Pra

THE WELLNESS-EMPOWERED WOMAN

"Reena's own journey through self-discovery to lead a balanced life and prioritizing her mental and physical health is truly inspiring. *The Wellness-Empowered Woman* is full of helpful takeaways and is a great reference guide that I can continue to use whenever I am in need of rebalancing!"

— **Meredith Momoda**, Vice President, Creative Partnerships at NBC Universal and Former Executive at Disney, Yahoo, Discovery Communications, and Oprah Winfrey Network

"Brava to Reena for her rallying cry to "keep moving." Finding my sacred place in the ballet studio as a lifelong hobby amplified my "passion and purpose" from the workplace to the boardroom. Everyone should read this playbook for stimulating your real passions and empowering your life."

— **Bonita Stewart**, Vice President, Global Partnerships at Google and Co-Author of *A Blessing: Women of Color Teaming Up to Lead, Empower and Thrive*

"In *The Wellness-Empowered Woman*, Reena addresses a unique cross-section of personal and professional development, empowerment, and wellness at a time when these tools are more needed than ever. This book will fill you with ideas about how to transform your life."

— **Jennifer Dulski**, CEO and Founder at Rising Team, Author of Purposeful and Former Executive at Facebook, Change.org, Google, and Yahoo

"Reena's passion for fitness is infectious, and her ideas for staying happy and healthy are ones that any equally busy working mom can use to instantly enrich her life. Her advice is the kind you want to and can act upon immediately—and it's most welcome at this time when mental and physical fitness have taken a backseat to work and family."

— **Meredith Bodgas**, Lead Editor at Toptal, Former Editor-in-Chief at *Working Mother Magazine* and Former Editor for *Hearst, Condé Nast,* and *Bauer*

"Reena Vokoun knows how challenging it is to try to do it all. Her heartfelt, personal story of awakening and transformation shows positive change is possible. Reena offers powerful reflection questions that invite us to consider choices and options that could transform our chaotic lives into more balanced, healthy and empowered lives. Reena is the coach and cheerleader we wish we all had."

— **Mary Oleksy**, Women in Management Groups Program Manager and Associate Director for Strategy and Curricular Support, Stanford Graduate School of Business

"It's become common advice to 'follow your passion,' but no one really explains what that looks like in a practical sense. And sure, we all know we're supposed to eat better, drink more water and get more sleep in an effort to live a happier, healthier life, but where does that fit into our over-worked, over-scheduled lives? In *The Wellness-Empowered Woman,* Reena Vokoun expertly weaves her own experience into actionable steps in each chapter to help any woman achieve her own personal best. As a busy woman trying to balance her career, marriage and motherhood, Reena has the relatable voice of a friend sitting next to you in a coffee shop. Her advice is nonjudgmental and acknowledges that we're all just trying to do our best while also giving us the tools we need to start feeling more fulfilled. *The Wellness-Empowered Woman* is a must-read for every woman out there tired of trying to be everything to everyone."

— **Kristi Dosh**, President and Publicist at Guide My Brand, Author of *Saturday Millionaires* and Former ESPN Sports Business Reporter

"Everyone talks about work/life balance, integration, or some variation of leading a life where your heart, mind, body and soul feel connected and aligned. While this is easy to say, it is so much harder to do. Reena writes a supremely practical guide for bringing things together, and she does it without judgment. Speaking from personal experience, she guides the reader through actionable steps to examine your life as it is today, imagine how it could evolve to be healthy and nourishing in every sense, and then help you get from here to there. This is a fantastic read for anyone, especially if you're experiencing burnout, stress, or another blocker to living your best life."

— **Lexi Reese**, Gusto COO and Former Executive at Google, Facebook, and American Express

THE WELLNESS-EMPOWERED WOMAN

LIVING A PASSION FIT LIFE TO ELEVATE YOUR HEALTH, HAPPINESS, FAMILY, AND CAREER

REENA VOKOUN

FUCHSIA ROSE
MEDIA

The Wellness Empowered Woman™: Living A Passion Fit Life to Elevate Your
Health, Happiness, Family, and Career
Published by Fuchsia Rose Media™
San Diego, CA

Publisher's Cataloging-in-Publication data

Names: Vokoun, Reena, author.
Title: The wellness empowered woman : living a passion fit life to elevate your
health , happiness , family, and career / Reena Vokoun.
Description: Includes bibliographical references. | San Diego, CA: Fuchsia Rose
Media, 2021.
Identifiers: ISBN: 978-1-7363647-0-3 (paperback)
Subjects: LCSH Self-actualization (Psychology.) | Self-realization. | Self-esteem. |
Self-esteem in women. | Self-confidence. | Self-confidence in women. | Success. |
Success in business. | Happiness. | Self-care, Health. | Women–Health. | Physical
fitness for women. | BISAC SELF-HELP / Personal Growth / Success | SELF-
HELP / Personal Growth / Happiness
Classification: LCC HQ1206 .V65 2021 | DDC 646.70082–dc23

Cover and Interior Design by Victoria Wolf
Book Cover and Author Headshot Photography by Alex Johnson

QUANTITY PURCHASES: Schools, companies, professional groups, clubs, and
other organizations may qualify for special terms when ordering quantities of this
title. For information, email contact@fuchsiarosemedia.com.

FUCHSIA ROSE
M E D I A™

To all the women across generations and around the world who aspire to transform their lives and make a positive impact—this book is for you, as we unite in friendship, sisterhood, and wellness.

CONTENTS

INTRODUCTION

MY
STORY

IN DECEMBER 2012, my life was in the early stages of a major transformation. The interesting thing is, I didn't quite know it yet.

At the time, a lot was going on in my life externally, and, at first, I was too busy to realize that something was happening internally. Although I felt stressed out, numb, powerless, unmotivated, lacking passion, and yearning for change, I didn't realize that something inside me was dying. The feelings I was experiencing, and my eventual realization of them, were the precursors for what was to come. Little did I know, a huge change and major rebirth would be forthcoming in the years ahead.

During this time in late 2012, I was a busy working mom of two boys who were five and almost two years old. Both my husband and I worked for Google in the fast-paced world of Silicon Valley, which created the dichotomy of a recognized privilege and a source of stress. We were ridiculously busy trying to manage our careers and our two active, energetic, and rambunctious little boys. We were going through the transition from preschool to kindergarten for our older son, potty training for our younger son, and trying to keep both of them happy, engaged, and out of trouble. Life was pure chaos!

My husband worked about eighty to a hundred hours a week and traveled 70 percent of the time. So I was often left to manage my work, the kids, and household by myself—while trying to hang on to my sanity! I worked about fifty to sixty hours a week and traveled about 25 percent of the time, which was one more challenge for us to manage.

Between both of us, we were continuously in meetings or on conference calls, working toward project deadlines, and traveling for work. Then, we came home and played with the kids; made dinner and cleaned up; performed bath, story, and bedtime routines; followed by more work at night. Our plates were overflowing daily. But, given our Type A personalities, can-do attitudes, and strong work ethics, we both thought we could handle it all. We also felt a sense of gratitude and passion for our careers and family. And, to be totally candid, we didn't feel we had a choice because everyone around us in Silicon Valley was working just as hard due to the intense tech industry work culture, competitive schools, and high real estate prices. We assumed this was the norm within the world we lived in.

In order to maintain our work and family responsibilities, my husband and I worked late and got up early. Neither of us slept well, and we started to develop insomnia. Since we were both so exhausted, our workouts started to go out the window, and we often found ourselves eating whatever leftover scraps the kids didn't finish, frequently ordering out, and not paying attention to the impact these bad habits were having on our health.

This fast-paced lifestyle started to catch up with us, and we both began to experience high stress, anxiety, and severe burnout, which weakened our immune systems and resulted in additional health issues. For example, I experienced chronic sinus infections and allergy-induced asthma, which continued on for years. Even today, it can flare up if I don't properly manage my health, allergies, immune system, and stress levels.

Because it was an extremely tough time for us, our kids, unfortunately, began to absorb all of our stress, which we noticed through their often defiant behavior and fights with each other to seek our attention in negative ways. During this time, I also developed some serious working mom's guilt, and I felt like I was totally failing as a mom because my mind was so preoccupied with keeping our ship afloat and not dropping any of the many balls I had in the air at work and at home.

Overwhelmed, my husband and I felt like we were on a crazy roller-coaster ride that we just couldn't get off of! We talked about the challenges we were facing but ultimately kept going because we didn't want to let anyone down, including our family, friends, employer, or each other. We became so wrapped up in our day-to-day struggles and our desire to do our best that we lost perspective.

I would often lie awake at night and think about how we got to this place. I reminisced about the exciting and amazing early years in our marriage when we both worked hard at the office and were on our laptops side by side at night but still had time to go to the gym, go out to dinner, and spend quality time together in the evenings and on the weekends. I also remembered the joy I felt when each of our sons was born and how much we enjoyed our precious family time together when I was on maternity leave and my husband was on paternity leave. I reminisced about how much I had always valued my health and well-being throughout my childhood, teenage, and adult years and how disciplined I used to be about exercising, getting enough sleep, eating healthy, and managing my stress. What happened? Where did I fall short? How did I get so lost along the way?

I'd always been a passionate person and put my heart and soul into everything I did, especially for the people and things that were near and dear to my heart. I'd had a lifelong passion for health, wellness, fitness, dance, mindfulness, and nutrition. I'd been trained in dance since the age of seven, I'd been teaching fitness classes since the age of eighteen, and I'd loved preparing and eating nutritious and healthy foods. These elements of health and wellness had always been a constant part of my life, but I became too busy to enjoy and participate in them once I became a working mom of one and then two children, while also trying to balance my career, family, and household.

Not only did I stop prioritizing my wellness practices during this time, but I also set aside the very tools I'd used my entire life to manage stress. As a first-generation-born Indian-American, I was introduced to yoga and meditation from my parents and grandparents at a very early age, since both are an integral part of the Indian culture and Hindu religion. These practices have always made me feel calm and centered. I'm grateful for this important element of my upbringing and consider it to be a gift and blessing in my life. However, as I focused on the pursuit of my corporate career while simultaneously growing my family, I barely used them, which led to my overwhelm and burnout.

In 2014, my maternal grandfather, my last living grandparent, the biggest supporter of me pursuing an entrepreneurial career in health and wellness, and the one who had inspired me through his entrepreneurial pursuits later in his career, passed away from heart disease—on my birthday. For a long time after his death, I was incredibly heartbroken, but I knew in my heart that he would have wanted me to get my and my family's health and life back on track and pursue my passions and dreams.

Long before my grandfather passed away, I often dreamed about leaving my corporate career, having more flexibility for my family and myself, and starting my own health and wellness company. But it seemed like a crazy thought at the time. Who would be foolish enough to walk away from an amazing company like Google and throw away her years of solid work experience with other Fortune 500 companies, including GE, CNET, Reebok, and Yahoo? And how could I deny that I did love the exciting world of digital advertising and media and my job at Google?

On top of that, I had worked hard in college at the University of Wisconsin–Madison and graduate school at Boston University. Wouldn't all that hard work go to waste if I suddenly changed careers? As a child of immigrant parents from India who worked so hard to provide a solid future for my brothers, sister, and me and who deeply valued education and stable careers, this was a decision I couldn't and didn't take lightly. What would my team and boss at work think? What would my parents, family, and friends think? What would my husband think? *What would I think?*

One night, despite my fears and worries, I started to visualize what I would name my company if I ever got the courage to start it. Then I had an epiphany and instantly came up with the name "Passion Fit," which I thought was such a powerful name and embodied me as a person. Was it potentially ... my future brand?! It was a life-changing moment and one I'll never forget. I felt a rush of excitement and hope, and I knew in my heart that I really wanted to make this dream a reality. So over the next few days, I came up with a tagline: "Pursue your passions, be fit and the rest will follow." It spoke to me deeply in terms of what I wanted to get back to in my life.

I had lost sight of these values during one of the most stressful times in my life, and it's ironic that I had a wake-up call with the loss of my sweet grandfather. I was able to find my way back to wellness through a lot of deep self-reflection, journaling, and talking with my loved ones. Through these efforts, I knew I was getting back to myself because I began to feel more optimistic and hopeful ... and in many ways, a new and improved self was beginning to emerge.

Ultimately, after two years of experiencing so much stress while also contemplating, planning, and dreaming of a career change, everything came to a head in 2014. I still remember the exact moment when I knew in my heart it was time to move on. We were in a team meeting to discuss the restructuring of our department to better meet client needs. Up until that point, I had been managing a portfolio of strategic partnerships in the publishing and entertainment industries on the West Coast, and based on the new structure, I would now be expanding my portfolio to a national level. I knew that expansion would mean more travel across the country for me, which at that point in my life, wouldn't have been sustainable. I also knew if I didn't make the change at that time, when would I ever do it?

My decision became clear. Although it was one of the biggest risks I'd ever taken and one of the most difficult decisions I'd ever faced, I finally made the bold and courageous move to leave Google. Thankfully, when I shared my desire to leave, I was met with tremendous support from my management team, colleagues, family, friends, and husband, especially when they saw the level of passion and conviction I had around having more flexibility for my family, launching Passion Fit, and wanting to help others.

Once I made the leap, I was able to have more time and space to think about how I wanted to design my life and balance the needs of my family, myself, and my new career. My life suddenly became different in every possible way. I began to live according to my values, which gave me freedom and control over my schedule and destiny, the ability to enjoy quality time with my family, and the opportunity to take better care of myself.

Even though I was now working hard from home to get my company off the ground, my kids seemed happier and more relaxed because I was around more. And my husband finally overcame his own burnout and ended up taking a different job at Google with better work-life balance. He and I were then able to deeply reconnect after going through such a difficult period in our lives. I finally felt alive again and excited for the future.

Looking back at my life before I began Passion Fit brings tears to my eyes—not only because of the recollection of the struggles I went through, but also because of the growth, life lessons, and deep and burning desire I have within me to share my experiences in order to help others who might also be struggling. And now, having written *The Wellness-Empowered Woman* in the midst of a global pandemic, economic crisis, social issues, climate change, and political upheaval, I feel even more strongly about sharing my authentic thoughts and insights to help provide empathy, hope, and optimism for a better future for us all. My intention through sharing what I've come to understand is to remind you that you're not alone, and wherever you are on your life's journey, change and transformation can happen for anyone, at any time, and at any stage in life.

CHAPTER 1

LIVING A PASSION FIT LIFE

MY COMPANY, PASSION FIT, is more than just a business. To me, it's a way of life. So what does it mean to live a Passion Fit life? To answer that, we need to start with the motto: "Pursue your passions, be fit and the rest will follow."

From my perspective, when you pursue things you're passionate about, it allows you to feel nourished and fulfilled. You're able to connect or reconnect with a deep part of yourself that makes you feel creative, vibrant, alive, and filled with purpose. You don't necessarily have to turn your passions into your career in the way I did ... unless you want to, of course! However, you can invite your passions into your life in other ways; for instance, taking classes, joining organizations, working on side hustles and projects, or engaging in anything else that fits into your interests and schedule.

For example, I have clients who are passionate about tennis and play on competitive women's tennis leagues, and other clients who are passionate about dance and have danced with performance troops. I also have clients who are passionate runners and train for 5K and 10K races, half marathons, and marathons every year, as well as clients who are passionate bloggers, photographers, poets, and artists, who have created businesses or content in these artistic areas. These clients are definitely living a Passion Fit life by enjoying their passions and activities, which adds a richness and depth to their lives in other areas too. They're more fulfilled, more confident, and have more energy to put into their jobs, families, and communities.

Before I launched Passion Fit, I started out by creating a blog and writing about health and wellness topics I was passionate about. My blog was intended to be the first step in getting my writing out into the public and to help prepare me to become an author down the road. I also launched my YouTube channel at that time and started working with a video production team in Silicon Valley to create health, wellness, and fitness video content.

I was doing all of this while still working for Google and tending to two young children. Yes, it was a crazy busy time, but honestly, those side projects lit a fire in me, gave me life, and solidified my desire and plans to launch Passion Fit several months later. I've always loved being able to express myself through writing and speaking, and throughout my career, I've also enjoyed working in digital media. So, it was fun and rewarding to begin creating my blog and video content around topics I'm passionate about in order to share my experiences, research, tips, and expertise with others.

The next part of the Passion Fit motto is to be fit. However, being fit isn't just in the physical sense. It's also in the mental, emotional, and spiritual sense, and together, I often refer to these as the four pillars of wellness.

If you eat nutritious foods and stay consistently active by making fitness an important part of your life, you'll inevitably have more energy, become stronger, increase your stamina, and prevent or manage diseases like diabetes and heart disease. Also, exercise allows you to release endorphins, which stabilizes your mood and is good for your mental and emotional health.

Practicing mindfulness is an essential part of being fit. It can positively impact your brain chemistry, stress levels, and spiritual outlook by allowing you to stay present-focused on your breathing and deeply connect with yourself. Having a positive mindset can help motivate you, allow you to be more productive, and help you take on challenges and setbacks and become more resilient and successful.

For most of my life, I've valued being fit through healthy eating, fitness, and mindfulness, but as I described in the introduction, I, unfortunately, lost sight of these tools when my stress levels were at their peak. I possibly could have prevented the burnout I experienced, or at least I could have better managed it, had I prioritized using these tools back then. However, I certainly learned a valuable lesson through that experience. No matter how busy, stressful, or overwhelming life gets, being able to stay fit in all these ways allows me to get through the tough times and come out flourishing in the end. In order for me to constantly remind myself of these lessons, I've built daily practices of meditation, yoga, exercise, healthy eating, and proper sleep into my life by blocking out time for these activities in my calendar every day and tracking them on my wearable device.

The last part of the Passion Fit motto states that if you pursue your passions and are holistically fit, the rest will follow—and I truly believe that. Since you'll be meeting your own needs, you'll be better equipped to meet the needs of your family, friends, employer, and community, and you'll be able to be of service to others. You'll be able to take on whatever comes your way because you invest in your own happiness and well-being and consistently take the time to care for yourself physically, mentally, emotionally, and spiritually. My own outlook on life certainly has evolved over the last several years of trials and tribulations, and I now have gained the wisdom and resilience to view every situation, both personal and professional, as an opportunity to learn, grow, and get better each day.

Finally, living a Passion Fit life means you already are or seek to become part of a supportive community that "gets you." Our Passion Fit community encompasses women from all over the world, with different careers, goals, challenges, family lives, personal lives, personalities, and backgrounds. My personal circle of friends, family, neighbors, school community, charitable community, and professional network (many of whom are also part of the Passion Fit community) are every bit as diverse and wonderful. However, one thing that connects everyone in my world is the fact that we all value being empowered through wellness in various ways, we all want to be the best we can be for others and ourselves, and we all greatly value our connections and relationships. These are the fibers of life that give it meaning and richness, and I believe having a community, or multiple communities, in your life can allow you to feel connected and supported to be at your best.

In *The Wellness-Empowered Woman*, I invite you to go on a journey to rediscover yourself or perhaps discover yourself for the first time. It's possible to flourish from the inside out, both personally and professionally, through wellness, so you can live a Passion Fit life filled with love, joy, peace, happiness, gratitude, and success. My desire is to guide you as a trusted friend and confidant on this exciting and life-changing adventure ahead.

Life is never perfect, and stress is inevitable. A big part of my learning and relearning was the need to have healthy tools to deal with whatever came my way. I will share with you the tools and practices that have become essential to my life, along with stories and examples based on my work with hundreds of clients of different races, ethnicities, life stages, careers, and backgrounds. I've included the latest research and stats on consumer and employee wellness, along with fresh tools that are holistic and focus on physical, mental, emotional, and spiritual well-being. I also provide innovative tips that include my Eastern and Western perspectives and philosophies, health and wellness tips for you and your families, and helpful resources for continued personal and professional development that support you and the communities and organizations you serve.

As we move into the next several chapters of the book, we're going to start to get more in depth about how you can live a Passion Fit life and become a wellness-empowered woman, as the two go hand-in-hand. They can give you the ability to banish burnout and step into your power with confidence and trust in yourself. You'll also gain more energy, optimize your health, and enhance your relationships. And finally, you'll have the tools to take your career to the next level, pursue your passions, experience new adventures, and enjoy your life to the fullest. So, get ready to dive into the content, grab a journal, and then answer the questions offered at the end of each chapter. The questions are an opportunity for you to pause and reflect so that you can start to make monumental changes in your life to succeed both personally and professionally through wellness, beginning right now.

QUESTIONS

1. What does pursuing your passions mean for you?

2. What does it mean to you to be "fit" in various aspects of your life?

3. How does participating in activities you're passionate about impact you mentally, physically, emotionally, and spiritually?

4. What does the concept of "the rest will follow" mean to you?

5. Where do you hope your transformation in these areas will lead you?

CHAPTER 2

WHAT'S YOUR GUT TELLING YOU?

WHEN YOU'RE IN A PERIOD OF TRANSITION or contemplating change or transformation, you may often hear the advice, "Listen to your gut" or "Trust your intuition." While these pieces of advice may sound like clichés, they actually can be invaluable in most situations, and your "woman's intuition" is an especially powerful tool you can tap into on a regular basis.

According to a study on the connection between intuition and mindfulness by the University of Hildesheim and featured in a June 9, 2015, *Psychology Today* article entitled "When Should You Trust Your Intuition?" by Susan Krauss Whitbourne, PhD, intuition can be particularly helpful in stressful and complex situations, such as managing career transitions, balancing work and family, organizing competing priorities, dealing with a lack of confidence, and being fearful of the past. If you're experiencing these types of situations, listening to your gut can give you a sense of self-awareness and a chance to honestly assess where you are in your life today.

However, in our extremely analytical data-driven world, we often shy away from listening to our gut, our deepest feelings, and our longings. Instead, we go crazy gathering data and then overanalyze, rationalize, and just plain talk ourselves out of what we may be truly feeling or wanting. Have you ever done this? I know I have. Why do we do this to ourselves? Well, we may not have the time to address our feelings because we're so busy, or we may not have the emotional capacity to deal with them because they're just too heavy, or we may be fearful of the outcome if we choose to address them. The problem is, if we continue to suppress these feelings and ignore any red flags or warning signs in our lives, the issues we're facing may snowball into something bigger. And then they could become serious and much more challenging to address.

It took me a while to listen to my gut and make the changes I wanted to make in my life because of my own fears, insecurities, worries about what others would think, and pure exhaustion at that time. In fact, it took me two whole years to experience an evolution in my behavior, where I recognized the signs of burnout, stopped overanalyzing myself and my situation, started making changes, and finally gained the courage and strength to leave my corporate career and start my own company.

While it was an extremely difficult decision, it was necessary and completely worth the risk. Once I made the decision, I knew in my heart it was the right one for my family and me. I honestly can't even imagine not making that decision and not living my life and running my career the way I am today. And had I kept going on the previous path I was on, who knows where my health, relationships, and career would be right now! I don't think I would be as healthy, happy, and fulfilled.

One of my clients had her own struggle with listening to her gut. She was feeling guilty that she had been working a lot and didn't have as much time to spend with her kids and spouse as she would like. She was up against several deadlines at work and was being considered for a promotion, and the decision was between her and a male colleague. She felt the pressure to be on her A-game at work, but her heart was hurting because her kids could feel she was stressed and preoccupied, and she'd recently missed yet another one of their school events. She rationalized with herself that this was only temporary, and once she got the promotion, she would be able to spend more time with her family. But would she?

If she did get that promotion, she likely would need to work more, not less. While she and her career were extremely important, it was critical for her to think of her career as a marathon and not a sprint. If she kept working at this crazy pace, she might end up burning out even more than she was already, missing more opportunities to be with her family, and possibly decreasing her chances of getting the promotion.

In this situation, it was best for her to slow down, take a deep breath, and tap into her intuition to see that she needed more balance and to build in more time for her family and herself. After not listening to her gut for so long, when she finally did, she was able to pay attention to her innermost feelings of guilt for not being around enough, her longing for more time with her family, and her anxiety about whether or not she would get the promotion. Also, she was able to give herself permission to take some breaks along the way, since she was stressed and tired. Taking those breaks helped her realize what her intuition was telling her all along: if that promotion was meant to be, it would happen without her need to sacrifice every aspect of her life to get it.

In the end, she got the promotion, and during the consideration process, she was able to figure out how to continue to listen to her inner voice, tune into the needs of herself and her family, and not run herself into the ground moving forward. By clearly communicating and setting boundaries in her personal and professional life, as her intuition was telling her to do, she was able to take on the promotion and approach her new position in a sustainable and healthy way. She eliminated the need to walk away from a beneficial advancement after all her hard work to earn it, and she decreased the possibility of creating more burnout or more issues at home.

Although these specific examples demonstrate what can happen when you listen to your intuition, it's important to consider what can happen when you don't. As described above, you might experience severe burnout, serious health problems, family issues, low performance at work, or other negative impacts that could create despair and lifelong regrets. In an effort to prevent the latter from happening, I invite you to take some time to listen to your own intuition. You know yourself better than anyone, which is why, as you step into becoming a wellness-empowered woman, you'll be able to fully trust yourself and your feelings. Here are five tips to begin "trusting your gut":

1. Be aware of your physical and emotional reactions and symptoms.

When we're faced with different decisions and situations in life, usually we have physical and emotional reactions, whether we're aware of them or not. For example, if a decision or situation seems to be in line with our values, needs, and wants, usually we feel calm, relaxed, and at peace. We have a normal resting heart rate and an easier time staying focused on the present. However, if we're feeling unsure about a decision or situation, are at a crossroads, or are feeling confused, our physical and emotional reactions may be different. They'll likely turn into stress. And according to 2017 Stress Statistics from the American Psychological Association, reported by *The American Institute on Stress*, 77 percent of people experience actual symptoms caused by stress. These symptoms could include:

- Rapid heart rate
- Headaches
- Increased blood sugar
- Insomnia
- Stomachache
- High blood pressure

- Weakened immune system
- Anxiety
- Depression
- Moodiness
- Feeling overwhelmed
- Fears from the past or for the future
- Difficulty concentrating
- Avoiding others

If you're experiencing any of these symptoms of stress, note what your gut is trying to tell you. These are warning signs or red flags you shouldn't ignore and are there to indicate something isn't quite right. Try to tune into your body and emotions, as they can provide insights to help you listen to your intuition and navigate different decisions and situations. Perhaps by journaling or talking to a loved one or professional about what you're feeling physically, mentally, and emotionally, you can pinpoint the root causes of why you're feeling the way you are and what your gut is trying to tell you to do or not do. The more you can practice this type of self-awareness, the easier it will become to do it, no matter what comes your way. You'll feel more confident and capable.

2. Take note of your immediate responses.

When you were in school, did your teachers ever tell you to go with your immediate or first response when answering questions on a test? This is basically trusting your gut or listening to your intuition. Oftentimes, we know more than we think we do because our brains are constantly encoding and storing information based on past learnings and experiences. We may not even realize all of the information that's there, but when we're faced with a question, we may have an immediate response or recall of that information, which comes to us at the moment we need it. In this same vein, when contemplating decisions or changes in your life, think about what your immediate response would be, because it will give you a good sense of the direction that might make the most sense for you.

As an example, let's say you and your sister want to train together for a triathlon. When she initially asks you to do it, your first response is yes, and you think it would be a fun challenge to take on. You're a decent runner and can ride a bike pretty well, but you may need to improve your swimming skills a bit. Nonetheless, you're ready to sign up, but the more you talk to your family and friends, the more they warn you and your sister about the risks involved, such as pointing out that it may be too strenuous, you both may get injured, you're too old, or you're not in good enough shape. You then start to doubt yourself based on everyone else's fears and reservations. However, at the end of the day, it's your and your sister's choice, and if you disregard your immediate response, you may regret it later. Your brain has likely stored a lot of information that led to your immediate response, and that's definitely worth paying strong attention to.

If your initial response was yes, there's a reason for that. Participating in the triathlon could be an amazing growth and bonding experience for both of you, and if you train properly, take it at your own pace, focus on safety, and prepare for all the challenges and opportunities that lie ahead, then why not? Go for it!

3. Think about what advice you would give to someone else in your situation.

Oftentimes, when we look at situations in our own life with someone else in mind, we may give advice that we might not always take ourselves. For example, it can be easy for us to tell our girlfriends, spouse, or parents how important it is for them to exercise and practice self-care. However, when it comes to ourselves, we may put our own needs for exercise and self-care on the back burner because we're so busy prioritizing and taking care of everyone and everything else.

Why is that? Do we think we don't deserve to take care of our own health through regular exercise and self-care too? Of course not. However, I've seen this happen too often with women, including myself in the past. If you're in the same boat, I want to invite us all to not put ourselves last. We'll only be left feeling depleted and resentful.

I come from a long line of women in my family who are caretakers and who consistently put everyone else's needs above their own. While this is partially a remnant of traditional Indian cultural norms and expectations, it's also commonplace for many women across the world today. As a result, I've done this throughout much of my adult life, especially after becoming a wife and mom—and often it's been at the expense of my own health and well-being.

However, over time, I've learned how critical it is to take my own advice and prioritize my needs as well. So now, when I start to neglect them and feel depleted and resentful, I remind myself that no one else will prioritize my needs for me; I have to do it for myself. Then, I communicate to my family that I need a break, and I take one to recharge through a good workout and sweat session, a hot shower, or whatever I need to take care of myself.

I encourage you to do the same. And as it relates to listening to your gut, take your own advice and trust what you feel inside. Again, if you're likely to give others advice based on what's in their best interest, make sure you do the same for yourself because you absolutely deserve it!

4. Pay attention to your dreams at night.

Dreams can be a powerful resource when trying to listen to your gut. According to a January 8, 2018, *Psychology Today* article written by Kelly Bulkeley, PhD, entitled "Intuition and Dreams: Four Questions to Ask of Each Dream," dreams are a natural source of intuition and insights. They can help tap into your subconscious mind and may provide clues to help you answer questions you might be struggling to answer.

While we often have strange or unexplainable dreams, such as falling, being chased, or getting lost, we don't necessarily have to take them at face value. Instead, we can look at the key themes, characters, emotions, and parallels to reality to try and make sense of them.

In an interview with *NBC News BETTER*, Robert Stickgold, PhD, associate professor of psychiatry at Harvard Medical School's Center for Sleep and Cognition, shared that during dreams at night, the brain tries to process and solve problems that were going on during the waking hours but weren't yet completed. This can be powerful information toward tapping into your intuitive thoughts and gut reactions to situations. It may also mean your unfinished business from the day is being brought into the forefront of your subconscious mind during your dreams at night, so you can find solutions over time.

After I left Google to start Passion Fit, I kept having recurring dreams that I decided to go back, and I would see myself back at the office in meetings with my former team. These dreams often were so vivid that I'd wake up in the morning and think I was back at Google! At first, I felt defeated and thought maybe it was a sign that I made the wrong decision by leaving the digital media industry, and it wasn't going to work out.

I did go through a brief period when I worked with a health and wellness technology start-up company in addition to running Passion Fit, as I thought I would gain more industry experience, and I could pursue both in parallel. I also had a few conversations with former colleagues and managers at Google about potentially coming back in the future. In the end, I decided to stick with my original plan to focus full-time on Passion Fit.

Over time, I've realized these dreams are simply a reminder of where I was and where I am now. I know in my gut that launching Passion Fit was the best decision for my career. I still use my digital media skills within my own company, and I'm happy with the impact I've made so far.

If you've had any recurring or vivid dreams about your personal or professional life, I encourage you to write them down as soon as you wake up, so you don't forget them. Try to be as descriptive and detail-oriented as you can. Who was in the dream? Where did it take place? Was the dream about a positive or negative situation? Was there a solution to a problem? How did you feel when you woke up?

Eventually, you may be able to distill key themes, patterns, people, challenges, or even outcomes. Then you can use this information to tap once again into your intuition, which may give you the ammunition you need to make a change or transformation in your life. With that, I want to wish you sweet dreams!

5. Look for signs all around you for validation.

Do you believe in using signs as guideposts in your life? I know for some, this may sound too kooky, spiritual, or intangible to believe in, but you can make it tangible by paying attention to words, objects, people, or other elements of your day-to-day life. The key is to have an open mind and heart and be willing to receive and analyze information that comes to you in new ways.

One of my clients knew she needed to exercise more, but she just couldn't find the time and motivation. However, when she went in for her annual physical, her doctor told her how critical it was to start working out more because her blood sugar was rising, and she was at risk of getting Type 2 diabetes. Shortly after her doctor's appointment, she saw a flyer for the studio where my Passion Fit classes were offered, which happened to be just a few miles from her house. She also saw the classes listed on Yelp and Facebook. Perhaps my marketing for Passion Fit just happened to reach her at the right time, but it also could have been a sign for her to start by taking classes and exercising more to improve her health and decrease her risk of getting Type 2 diabetes. Thankfully, she did take the classes and improve her numbers!

When I was in college studying business, I regularly taught fitness classes on campus and continued to train and perform in different styles of dance. While these were activities I simply did on the side, they were huge passions of mine. They stuck with me throughout my adult life, and no matter what else I had going on with work, college, or graduate school, I made time to teach fitness classes, dance, perform, and train for fitness competitions. While I didn't know then that these passions would become a part of my signature offerings for Passion Fit, signs were everywhere that they would continue to play a significant role in my life.

These types of scenarios happen all the time in our everyday lives. We just have to be awake and aware, paying close attention to what's happening all around us while thinking about why things happen the way they do. We may not understand what's happening in the present, but when we look back, situations may start to make more sense, as the signs were there all along. Whether or not you consider yourself to be a spiritual person, it's possible to tap into signs in your life. As you begin to focus on what's happening and why, you'll naturally become more present-focused and more perceptive and intuitive to yourself, others, and your environment. Life may also become more colorful, rich, and fulfilling.

Listening to your gut and following your intuition can

make all the difference in solving problems and making changes in your life. While gathering data and analyzing situations are important, it's more important to first listen to your deepest feelings and longings because they provide you with the real story. Usually, when we don't listen and we ignore our inner voice, it will find a way to keep coming back and try to alert and warn us. The key is to learn to listen to that inner knowing so you don't have to look back and wish you would have done it sooner.

In the days and weeks ahead, try to find time to become aware of your physical and emotional reactions, take note of your immediate responses, think about the advice you would give to others in your situation, pay attention to your dreams, and take note of signs happening all around you. The time to do these things is now. Your intuition is there, waiting for you to tap into it!

QUESTIONS

1. What does the concept of listening to your gut mean to you?

2. Can you think of a time when you listened to your gut as well as a time when you didn't? What happened in each instance?

3. Is there anything coming up in your life right now that might require you to tap into your intuition?

4. If so, how can you create space in your life to listen to your inner voice to make the best decision for you?

5. What is your desired outcome in this situation, and how can you make it a reality?

CHAPTER 3

BALANCE, INTEGRATION, OR WHATEVER YOU WANT TO CALL IT!

IN RECENT YEARS, there has been a lot of debate over whether work-life balance, especially for women and working moms, is even possible. For many, it seems like an elusive goal. As a result, many industry experts prefer to use the term "work-life integration." In my opinion, the term isn't as important as the understanding that we all need to figure out how to have both a personal and professional life and allow the two to coexist in ways that work for our loved ones, our employers or our own businesses, and ourselves.

Work-life balance, work-life integration, or whatever you want to call it, will look different for each person. As we continue this journey to become a wellness-empowered woman, we will look at how you might define what it looks like based on your core values, personal and family life, health considerations, career path, goals, inner desires, and other needs.

When I was pregnant for the first time with my older son, I was focused on figuring out how to have the "perfect work-life balance," and I was determined to make it happen and thrive. When my husband and I were newlyweds just a few years earlier, I had attended graduate school part-time while working in a full-time corporate job. As a result, I already had some experience with juggling and figuring out work-life balance, so I could handle it ... right? I definitely was still trying to figure out work-life balance back then and wasn't always successful at it, but I kept trying.

I regularly attended conferences for working moms (yes, they're really a thing), read countless books on working motherhood, and even subscribed to the magazine *Working Mother*, which, ironically, I now write for on a regular basis. Somehow, I thought if I put in the work to prepare before my baby arrived, I would be able to figure it all out and seamlessly balance my career and family life. In theory, it made sense, but in reality, boy was I wrong!

Organization and logistics aside, no one quite prepares you for what happens to your heart when you have a child. You can be the most ambitious, hardworking, and career-driven woman on the planet (and believe me, I was one of them and still am today!), but when you're blessed with a precious new baby in your life, that's when the internal conflict begins ... at least that's what happened to me.

I was fortunate enough to receive almost six months of maternity leave, which was such a blessing. But throughout that sweet and exhausting time at home, learning to be a mom, nursing, changing diapers, cooking, and taking care of household chores, while also enjoying glorious moments as a family and creating wonderful memories, I oftentimes looked at my adorable baby boy as I rocked and sang him to sleep at night and became stressed when I thought about what life would look like when it was time to go back to work.

I was working in digital advertising sales for Yahoo prior to and while on maternity leave, and while I enjoyed my job and knew I wanted to go back to work, I wanted more flexibility and needed to figure out, with my husband, what childcare would look like for our family. Yahoo didn't have a corporate daycare, and my request to come back to work part-time wasn't approved. While I understood and respected the decision, I was torn about what to do.

Around the same time, a recruiter reached out to me about an open business development and sales position in digital advertising at Google. While I was initially hesitant to switch jobs and companies right after having a baby and finishing up maternity leave, I was well aware that Google had a world-class corporate daycare. I also would be able to have a more flexible schedule if I came to work for Google, based on what the recruiter told me about the culture within the company and the team I would be interviewing to work with. So I went through the interview process and ended up getting a job offer. While I was sad to leave my wonderful team at Yahoo, I knew working at Google would be a great next step in my career, and I was excited about the corporate daycare for my son and having a more flexible schedule.

Although this arrangement seemed to be ideal for a working mom, I'll never forget those early days and months of dropping off my son at daycare and trying to balance my new responsibilities as a mom with my role as a new employee at Google. On the outside, I appeared to be fine and was able to pull it together at work, but on the inside, I was struggling … and I do partially blame postpartum hormones for that! I often cried before and after work because I felt so guilty for leaving my son. My mom was a stay-at-home mom, and back then, my brothers, sister, and I stayed home with her until each of us went to kindergarten. I wanted so badly to give my son what my mom had given my siblings and me, but deep down, I knew times were different, and I also still wanted to have a successful career like my dad.

Like all the other working moms before me and the many who have and will continue to come after me, I had to go through some growing pains, which required that I figure out what worked best for me and my family. Struggling, having victories, then more struggles, then more victories, and everything in between was part of the process for me to learn how to balance my career, family, and life. Over time, I began to figure things out, and it became easier to manage. With the establishment of Passion Fit, I ultimately found a better work-life balance for myself. Experience provides perspective,

perspective provides wisdom, and wisdom provides space for creative solutions and contentment. It was not a straight path to nirvana by any means ... but it was a worthwhile experience in which I had the opportunity to learn and grow and be better for it in the long run!

We all can do many things to better manage our personal and professional lives to create greater work-life balance and, in essence, become wellness-empowered women. In the upcoming chapters in this book, we'll cover specific topics, such as stress management, mindfulness, fitness, sleep, productivity, and nutrition. However, before we get to those topics, let's focus on having the right mindset around work-life balance.

According to an April 6, 2017, article by Eric Garton in *Harvard Business Review*, psychological and physical problems of burned-out employees cost between $125 billion to $190 billion a year in healthcare spending in the US. Burnout has become a serious problem, and in many cases, it has become an epidemic. When we're caught up in the daily grind of work, family, and life in general, we often lose sight of the bigger picture and may not even realize we're running ourselves into the ground. Most of the time, we're just trying to survive each day as best as we can.

However, consistently taking a step back and assessing our daily and/or weekly schedules, habits, moods, and emotions are essential if we want to protect our health and well-being. We need to be honest with ourselves and write down what's truly going on. If these elements of our lives aren't serving us well, we have to be willing to stop and figure out how to make changes. The more we can do this regularly, the less risk we have for letting our work and personal life get completely out of balance and out of control. It's up to each of us to have a mindset that supports taking stock of our own lives regularly because no one else will do it for us, including those in our personal life or professional network. So how do you do this, you ask? Well, here are three ideas to help you.

1. Schedule a weekly work-life balance review with yourself.

I know it might sound silly or too formal and rigid, but it's an effective way to create a consistent check-in and know where you stand. If your job is important enough for your boss to conduct a regular review with you or for you to conduct one if you have your own business, then you're important enough to conduct one for yourself, your health, and your level of work-life balance. It may be helpful to ask yourself the following list of questions every week, or you can create your own list. You can also update or change these questions as your life evolves.

- What does my schedule look like these days?
- Does my workload feel manageable right now?
- Am I spending enough time with my family?
- Am I making time to tend to my own needs?
- How is my health these days?
- How are my energy levels?
- How are my emotions?
- Are my habits healthy, or do I have any unhealthy habits I need to pay attention to?

- Do I feel I can thrive in my day-to-day life most days, or am I constantly in a state of exhaustion?
- If I could change anything in my life right now, what would it be?
- What do I need to do to make necessary changes or to keep things the way they are?

These types of questions allow you to dig deep and figure out where there may be issues. When life moves at lightning speed, as it often does, it can be difficult to slow down or even pause unless we build it into our life and force ourselves to do it.

2. Block time in your calendar for health, wellness, and family activities.

In order to be a wellness-empowered woman who strives to balance her personal and professional life, I highly recommend becoming best friends with your online calendar, and if you don't already have one, create one now. Trust me, it will not only save you from burning out, but it will actually help you thrive!

The key is to create consistency in how you label and color code meetings, appointments, events, and reminders. I do this religiously with my calendar, and it helps me stay organized and on track. For example, work meetings and deadlines are in bright green, volunteer activities are in red, self-care activities are in purple, activities for my kids and husband are in blue, and leisure, relaxation, and entertainment activities are in dark green. It really helps me to look at my day and see where I'm spending my time, what I need to accomplish, where I need to be, and when and where I need to make adjustments.

Your calendar is a wonderful mechanism to block out time for your health, wellness, and family needs, so it doesn't get overridden by work obligations. I try to be diligent about building time into my day for sleep, exercise, meditation, meals, self-care, relaxation, and family. That way, I'm more likely to prioritize these activities so my days and weeks don't get overrun by work.

However, please remember that everyone is different, so you'll want to find a system that works for you. If my system seems too rigid, detailed, or unsustainable, you can always simplify or change it. Find what works best for you, and then stay consistent with it. And if you need to evolve or change it over time to better meet your needs as your life changes, please feel free to do so.

3. Set expectations at work and home.

It's also critical to set expectations at work with your boss, team, and clients, along with your family at home. If you aren't clear about your schedule, abilities, boundaries, and limitations, everyone will expect as much out of you as they can possibly get. It's not intended to be malicious or inconsiderate; it's just the reality that when people feel they need you, they need you. If you're a people pleaser like me and many of my friends, family members, and clients, you'll want to pay extra attention to this section.

Sometimes we assume people can read our minds. I know so many women, including myself, who truly think our spouses, significant others, kids, employers, or business partners know when we're struggling, are frustrated, or just need a break. Now, some people, especially those who are really perceptive or highly emotionally intelligent, can see when we're in these challenging states, and I applaud them for that. My mom is one of those people for me, and oftentimes, my husband can be. The look on my face or the sound in my voice can be a dead giveaway for them, and then they'll ask me what's wrong or what I need in those moments. However, we can't expect this from the people in our lives all the time. They're only human and may have their own struggles they're dealing with.

I want to encourage you to set expectations at work and at home and clearly communicate what you need and when you need it from those in your life, especially on a day-to-day basis. Believe me, they will thank you for being honest and communicative because then they don't have to guess, wonder, or feel as if they've let you down. It creates a win-win for everyone when you say things to your employer, business partners, spouse, significant other, or kids, such as:

- "I'm pretty exhausted from finishing up that last big project and would appreciate a day to reset so I'll have the energy to take on the next one."
- "I'm going to take next Friday afternoon off work to take my kids shopping for school supplies. I'll be sure to manage my workload, client communications, and calendar accordingly."
- "I would appreciate some help with school drop-offs

and pickups for the kids this week because my plate is really full."
- "Let's plan a trip to the beach next weekend because I would love some relaxation time with the family."
- "I need you and your brother to please help me get the table set for dinner."
- "I need you and your sister to please listen to me and put your toys and bikes away."

These are clear and kind statements that allow you to let others know exactly what you need. If you had to put your own statement list together, what would it look like for you? The more we practice, the better we'll be at setting expectations, creating boundaries, and using clear communication to kindly make our voices heard and get our needs met. I believe these changes can make a big difference in your life!

Again, while work-life balance will hold different meanings for different people and at different stages of life, putting in the time to figure out what works for you is critical to achieving both personal and professional success and preserving your health and well-being in the process.

1. How do you define work-life balance?

2. While life is never perfect, how will you benefit if
    you focus more on creating this balance to the best
    of your ability on an ongoing basis?

3. How can you build a weekly work-life balance
    review into your life?

4. What health, wellness, and family activities can you
    start blocking time for in your calendar?

5. How can you better set expectations at work and
    at home?

CHAPTER 4

YOUR GENES DON'T HAVE TO DETERMINE YOUR JEANS

I'M FASCINATED BY THE CONCEPT OF epigenetics. In the book *Super Genes* by Deepak Chopra, MD, and Rudolph E. Tanzi, PhD, epigenetics is defined as having the ability to affect our own genome, which consists of our genetic material and DNA, through daily lifestyle choices, including diet, exercise, stress management, sleep, mindfulness, and self-care. No longer do we need to be victims of our genetic predispositions brought upon us by our ancestors. We truly have the power to diminish, manage, and potentially even conquer diseases and mental health challenges such as obesity, diabetes, heart disease, cancer, anxiety, and depression. Our genes don't have to determine the size of our jeans, or anything else for that matter!

While we can't do anything about the genes we were born with, we can silence the bad genes and turn up the good genes, so to speak, by designing and living our lives in a healthy, safe, and balanced way. Many examples demonstrate how lifestyle choices can allow us to do just that, which we'll cover in this chapter. The key is to first understand what we're up against in terms of our genetic predispositions, and then figure out what we need to do to prevent or manage them with the support of our healthcare practitioners and family. Everyone will have different focuses and priorities, and we each need to create a customized plan to manage our health and lifestyles accordingly.

I worked with a client who had breast cancer, which ran in her family. Thankfully, she was in remission and working with her doctors to prevent the cancer from coming back. She had to make some lifestyle adjustments along the way. For example, after treatment and recovery from breast cancer and after getting her doctor's clearance to exercise, I recommended she start with moderate levels of physical activity that didn't involve much upper body strength training work because her breast area, torso, arms, and hands were still tender and needed time to recover and get stronger. We prioritized low-impact cardio, dancing, walking, and light Pilates, which focused more on the core, back, and lower body to start. We also had to ensure her nutrition plan included a plant-based diet with an increase in vegetables, fruits, and whole grains, and a decrease in fats and artificial or processed foods. She had to ensure her alcohol intake was minimal and needed to manage her stress on an ongoing basis through mindfulness and breathing practices, which I shared with her. By making these lifestyle changes, she increased her chances of staying healthy and decreased her chances of a recurrence of cancer.

I've also worked with and personally know people who have avoided or overcome mental health issues in their DNA through tools such as regular meditation, exercise, and talking with a professional. Along with the help of their healthcare practitioners who prescribed Western and/or alternative medicines, where appropriate, they've been able to take control of their brain chemistry and mental health in order to live happy, healthy, and fulfilled lives.

Diabetes and heart disease run in my family, so I make daily decisions for my own health to ensure I can silence those genes. For example, I'm diligent about eating natural and plant-based foods and avoid or minimize my consumption of red meat, processed foods, and foods high in sugar, sodium, saturated fats, and trans fats. I also exercise daily to ensure I'm managing my weight, blood sugar, and cardiovascular health. Finally, I manage my stress levels through meditation, prayer, journaling, and talking to my husband, family, and close friends about challenges I may be facing. I also strive to get sufficient sleep on a regular basis.

To ensure our daily lifestyles are set up in the optimal way, it's important to talk openly with our parents and grandparents about the various diseases that run in our families and be proactive by getting the proper screenings and checkups at the appropriate ages in our lives so we can prevent or manage these diseases. Examples include getting regular mammograms for breast cancer, skin and mole checks for skin cancer, blood sugar tests in general and during pregnancy for both regular and gestational diabetes, EKGs and chest X-rays for heart disease, lung function tests for asthma, and food and environmental tests for allergies. It's better to find out about the potential risks and threats early on rather than late in the game or before it's too late. Awareness and action are critical and can mean the difference between surviving or thriving, and they can save your life.

So how can you apply the concept of epigenetics to your day-to-day life? As mentioned, first and foremost, study up on your family's health history so you have a thorough understanding of it. Next, talk to your healthcare practitioner and think about what lifestyle adjustments you'll want to make over time and then start to build out a plan. Tackle one key behavior change at a time to ensure the adjustments are realistic and sustainable.

According to B.J. Fogg, PhD, a behavior scientist at Stanford University and the author of the *New York Times* bestselling book *Tiny Habits*, behavior changes need three elements to be successful: (1) ability, (2) a prompt, and (3) motivation. Pick simple changes that are within your ability level; provide a prompt, at least at first, to encourage you to take the action; and then have the means to keep yourself motivated by positively reinforcing the changes you've made so that you'll want to carry them out each day. Once you hit about sixty-six days, which is approximately how long it takes for a behavior change to stick, it will hopefully become a healthy habit and a regular part of your daily life. Then you can move on to the next behavior change you want to tackle.

Let's look at a few examples. If obesity runs in your family and you're trying your best to prevent it in your thirties after having two kids, then you might want to make some behavior changes around your eating habits and nutrition plan. One change might include reducing your carbohydrate intake and only eating whole grains at breakfast and lunch and choosing not to include them at dinner. Your dinners could include foods rich in protein, vegetables, and fiber, such as chicken, fish, beans, lentils, broccoli, spinach, zucchini, and tomatoes, and would not include pasta, rice, bread, and the like. You would need to practice making this change on a certain day, and congratulate yourself for doing it, which will motivate you to do it again the next day, the day after that, and so on and so forth, until it becomes a healthy habit after about two months. Over time, you may lose weight or maintain your weight, depending on what you needed to protect against obesity.

Here's another example. Perhaps anxiety runs in your family, and you're feeling extra anxious because you're planning to transfer jobs within your company and will be moving to a new city. The thought of starting a new role is stressful enough, but the logistics of packing, physically moving, and having to start over in a place where you don't know anyone feels even more daunting. Before allowing your anxiety to get the best of you, you could start practicing yoga for thirty minutes a day by using a yoga app in the evenings at home to calm your mind and body and give you some perspective. You would apply the same behavior-change principles to finding a yoga practice that's easy to do and within your abilities, motivating yourself through positive reinforcement, and then doing it again and again. After slowing down and connecting with yourself on a regular basis, you would most likely have the ability to get your anxiety under control and be in a healthy mental state prior to your job transfer and move.

What I love most about the concept of epigenetics is the ability to have hope and focus on things we can control when it comes to our health, well-being, and life. While we may not always have complete control over what happens, especially when we may be dealing with strong genetic predispositions, we can still be as proactive as possible. There are also growing bodies of research, medical science, knowledge, and effective tools to help us live our healthiest lives possible, which is extremely encouraging, motivating, and empowering!

QUESTIONS

1. How do you feel about the concept of epigenetics?

2. What genetic predispositions do you have?

3. Have you talked with your family about the details around your family's health history and these genetic predispositions?

4. What are the most important lifestyle changes you need to make for disease prevention or management?

5. What's one behavior change you can start making today, and how can you execute it and stay motivated to keep doing it on an ongoing basis to protect your health?

CHAPTER 5

THE CALM BEFORE THE STORM?

HAVE YOU EVER ANTICIPATED AN EVENT or situation that seemed like it would be extremely stressful, but then when it actually happened, it wasn't so bad after all? Anticipation is often worse than reality, and anxiety is often caused by expecting the worst to happen. In many cases, the "calm before the storm," as the saying goes, doesn't actually change, and the storm never comes! In fact, according to a July 19, 2019, article in *Psychology Today* by Seth J. Gillihan, PhD, entitled "How Often Do Your Worries Actually Come True?" researchers at Penn State University did a study on this very topic, and it concluded that 91 percent of the worries were false alarms and never came true.

Now, I'm not saying anxiety isn't a serious mental health

condition, because for many people, it can be. According to the Anxiety and Depression Association of America, anxiety disorders are the most common mental health issues in the US and impact forty million adults each year. However, whether you experience mild or severe anxiety, in addition to seeking out professional and/or medical help if needed, practicing mindfulness can be an extremely helpful and effective tool for rewiring your brain chemistry to help you become more calm, relaxed, and clear-headed, even during challenging times. This chapter will show you how, based on my unique Indian-American upbringing and formal training in yoga and meditation.

Growing up as a first-generation-born Indian American, I've seen my parents practice meditation, yoga, and pranayama breathing on a near-daily basis, which they learned from my grandparents. Seeing multiple generations in my family leveraging these mindfulness tools has had a profound impact on me because I've seen firsthand how powerful they can be in naturally empowering and enhancing your life. These deeply rooted elements of the Indian culture and Hindu religion came into existence thousands of years ago, and for me, there's a sense of comfort and wisdom in adopting practices that have been around for such an extended period of time and have been scientifically proven to benefit humans.

According to research through Harvard Medical School, yoga and meditation can help reduce stress response systems often found in anxiety and can also change the structure of the brain. Hormones and chemicals such as serotonin, cortisol, and endorphins are released to promote a sense of calm, memory, focus, and learning. In addition, pranayama breathing helps to rid the body of toxins and promotes a flow of energy and oxygen throughout the body.

Over the years, I've attended countless yoga classes, have completed coursework and training to teach yoga and meditation, and still practice it a few times a week as part of my regular fitness and mindfulness regimen. I also enjoy lighting a candle, playing relaxing music, and simply sitting and centering myself through a focus on deep breathing. In addition, I enjoy using meditation apps and often include my kids and husband in my meditation sessions before bedtime. And finally, I like to incorporate meditation when I pray every day. It makes me feel spiritual, centered, and at times, even enlightened.

I encourage my clients to do yoga, meditation, and deep breathing, and I incorporate all three religiously in the different types of fitness and dance classes I teach. I have many clients who are working moms and often feel stressed, frazzled, and out of balance in their daily lives. In my classes, I want them to take time out of their busy lives to completely turn inward and focus on themselves. It's a chance to tune out the noise and chaos and strive to find quiet, peace, and tranquility. It's a little gift I'm able to give to them and they're able to give themselves, even if only for a few minutes in their day.

I've definitely had moments in my life when I've felt extremely stressed and anxious. One moment in particular was on Thanksgiving Day a few years ago. We were in the Midwest celebrating Thanksgiving with my in-laws. We had just arrived, and our kids were excited to play with their cousins. Immediately upon seeing each other, the kids all ran downstairs to the basement and started to engage in a game of tag. However, little did we know, they were playing in the dark, on the slippery floor, with only socks on their feet. Running fast, my younger son ended up slipping and hitting the side of his head on a water heater pipe.

My older son immediately ran upstairs and frantically told my husband and me what had happened, so we ran downstairs to find our younger son crying, with blood everywhere. I. Mean. Everywhere. I was in shock, and my heart was beating so fast that it felt like it was going to burst out of my chest. It was one of the most scary and anxious moments in my life. We grabbed some towels, applied them to our son's head, and asked him some questions to make sure he was conscious and still alert. He answered our questions through tears and was alert, but he was obviously scared and in a lot of pain. We raced to the car so we could take him to the ER.

He ended up having a deep cut on the side of his head, which required staples, as well as a moderate concussion. He had to keep the staples in for a little over a week to allow the cut to heal and wasn't able to play sports or do anything too strenuous at school for about eight weeks to allow the concussion to heal. Thankfully, he ended up okay, but our whole family will never forget that Thanksgiving Day experience.

In those moments when we all were feeling stressed and anxious, we needed to take long, deep breaths to calm our minds and bodies, which is what we did. We also prayed and kept reassuring our son and each other that everything would be okay. As a mom, it was imperative that I stay calm. I didn't want my son to be more worried than he already was—he was looking to me for comfort while my husband was handling the logistics of getting us to the ER and filling out paperwork once we got there. A tall order for sure, but a necessary one. Those mindfulness practices I learned from my parents came in handy in that difficult and scary moment. While my son's injury was serious, staying mindful and focused on the present prevented us from future-tripping or imagining the situation to be even worse than it was. And thankfully, he was able to heal and get back to normal within several weeks.

While mindfulness is an important tool to use during those dramatic and chaotic moments in our lives, we also can use it in everyday life. It's especially helpful to use mindfulness tools in everyday life because those practices prepare you for unexpected life situations, big and small, and give you the strength, courage, and wisdom to get through them. Thankfully, more and more people are realizing the importance of mindfulness. According to research conducted through the National Center for Complementary and Integrative Health, the number of US adults practicing meditation tripled between 2012 and 2017, and that number has only continued to increase over the last few years.

Whether you regularly practice mindfulness, have never tried it, or are somewhere in the middle, I want to share some ideas around yoga, meditation, and deep breathing that you can easily incorporate into your everyday life. It doesn't have to be intimidating or something you dread, and it actually can be really fun. You can even incorporate mindfulness practices when you're walking, hiking, or biking in nature, at the end of a workout, or before you go to sleep. My goal is to help you look forward to your mindfulness practices and treat them as an opportunity to create your own little peaceful sanctuary each day.

Yoga: Yoga came into existence five thousand years ago and is derived from the Sanskrit word "union." It combines mental, physical, and spiritual elements into one cohesive mind-body practice. If you're looking to incorporate this mind-body practice into your life, below are listed the twenty basic yoga poses that I incorporate into my own practice and in my classes. They are a combination of standing poses and poses on the mat. You can mix and match these poses and do them at the end of a workout or as a standalone activity in the morning before work, in the evening after work, in the middle of the day if you have the flexibility in your schedule, or at night before bedtime. You also can combine them together into a full vinyasa flow. Be sure to check with your healthcare practitioner before engaging in these poses if you have any injuries or health concerns. And if you need to see a visual of these poses, feel free to check out my yoga video series on the Passion Fit YouTube channel at youtube.com/passionfitllc.

1. Warrior I
2. Warrior II
3. Warrior III
4. Chair pose
5. Mountain pose
6. Tree pose
7. Standing bow pose
8. Plank pose

9. Chaturanga pose
10. Baby cobra pose
11. Cobra pose
12. Bow pose
13. Downward dog pose
14. Side plank pose (This is the graphic on the Passion Fit company logo!)
15. Child's pose
16. Pigeon pose
17. Cat cow pose
18. Boat pose
19. Butterfly pose
20. Shavasana pose

As you become more consistent with your yoga practice, you'll notice an energy flow between your mind and body. You'll also feel more mentally and physically strong and centered.

Meditation: The word meditation means to "focus" or "ponder," and the earliest practices of meditation stem from Hinduism. The goal of meditation is to achieve purification of the mind, body, and soul. In preparation to start practicing, find a quiet place and get into a comfortable position, either sitting cross-legged with your palms facing up and resting your hands on your legs or lying down with your arms at your side. You can have soft and calming music playing in the background (in the Indian culture, we usually listen to music with a sitar instrumental), or you can be in silence.

Close your eyes and start to focus on your breathing and

bringing your heart rate down. In the Indian culture, we also chant the word, "Om, shanti, shanti, shanti," which means peace, but that's optional. Relax your mind and body and let go of any tension in your muscles. Stay centered and try to only focus on the present moment and your breathing, clearing your mind of any other thoughts. If your mind starts to wander, don't judge yourself, and gently bring your attention back to your breathing and the present moment.

You can also incorporate positive visualization, where you picture your loved ones or a relaxing destination, such as a beach, waterfall, forest, mountain, or any other place that's calming and relaxing to you. Another option is to focus on positive affirmations, such as thinking to yourself that you're strong, wise, centered, and capable of handling anything that comes your way.

The key to meditation is to be kind to yourself, avoid any harsh judgments, and connect with your inner being. Being able to tune out what's happening in the outside world and pay attention to your own inner needs are key components of meditation. You can practice for as long as you want or need, and even practicing for as little as five minutes a day can make a huge difference in managing anxiety and caring for your mental, emotional, and spiritual health.

Breathing: Breathing is essential to human existence and is also critical for good physical and mental health. You can try different types of breathing, and you can incorporate them into your yoga and meditation practices.

One type is pranayama breathing, which involves breathing deeply through both nostrils, holding your breath for a second, and then slowly exhaling through your nose. You can also use your ring fingers and thumbs to push down on one nostril at a time while you take deep and short breaths through the other nostril.

Another type of breathing is diaphragmatic breathing, which involves expanding your belly and diaphragm as you inhale through your nose and then exhale through your mouth or nose as you pull your belly back in to a neutral position. It's a long and deep form of breathing, as opposed to shallow breathing through the chest, which can often cause you to hyperventilate and feel more stressed and anxious.

Finally, lateral breathing, which is often used in yoga and Pilates, involves keeping your core engaged, while directing your breath up and into your ribcage. You inhale through your nose and then exhale through your mouth or nose.

Regardless of what type of breathing technique you choose, you'll be able to improve the health of your lungs, lower your heart rate, allow oxygen and energy to flow through your body, and rid your body of toxins.

While life can certainly have its ups and downs with expected and unexpected situations, we have the power to control our awareness, reactions, actions, or inactions through mindfulness tools such as yoga, meditation, and deep breathing techniques. I encourage you to find ways to incorporate these tools into your day-to-day life, as they have the power to be life-changing!

QUESTIONS

1. Do you ever experience anxiety? If so, how does it make you feel and what do you do currently to calm yourself?

2. How do you feel about yoga?

3. How do you feel about meditation?

4. How do you feel about deep breathing techniques?

5. How can you incorporate these mindfulness tools into your day-to-day life?

CHAPTER 6

NO MATTER WHAT ELSE IS GOING ON, KEEP MOVING!

I'VE ALWAYS BEEN AN ACTIVE PERSON. I currently teach fitness and dance classes four to five days a week, and work out with my clients too. I also try to get in workouts on my own another one to two days a week and usually plan for at least one rest day a week. I find that this routine helps me to stay physically, mentally, emotionally, and spiritually healthy and able to manage my stress and be more productive.

According to the Harvard School of Public Health and countless other sources, exercise is one of the very best things you can do for your health. And according to the American Heart Association, regular exercise improves sleep, promotes a positive outlook, builds confidence and self-image, allows you to get outdoors, increases energy, and encourages social connection with others. Most of us already know this, but when life takes over, we can easily forget these essential benefits that can take us from being burned out and bitter to thriving and thankful.

Whether you're feeling stuck on a project at work, lethargic on the weekends, or anxious about your to-do list, getting your body moving can go a long way to improving your mood and ability to take action. This chapter is intended to inspire you and show you how to get started—or keep going—even if you get stuck along the way!

My love for movement began at the age of seven. I started taking ballet lessons and immediately fell in love with it. I continued with ballet throughout my childhood and also trained in other styles of dance during my teenage and adult years, including modern, hip hop, jazz, Bollywood, and Latin.

In high school, I was co-captain of my school's dance team and choreographed and co-led the team through competitions, in addition to performing at our high school basketball and football games. It was such a fun and rewarding experience, and I have very fond memories of that time in my life.

I then took dance classes for elective credits in college and also became a dance instructor at that time, where I worked with high school dance teams at summer dance camps. It was fun to share my knowledge and love of dance with others. With dance, there was and still is something powerful about being able to choreograph and master different routines by blending various movements, positions, and poses to create a sense of fluidity and tell a story, while moving the body in synchronicity with music and expressing oneself in an authentic way.

In addition to dance, I also became passionate about fitness at an early age. I discovered workout shows on ESPN, and I'd religiously do them after school throughout late elementary, middle, and high school. I joined a gym with my sister when I was in high school and started weight training. I was able to apply my dance skills to my workouts and really enjoyed building up my cardiovascular and strength-training capabilities, which, in turn, made me a stronger dancer and gave me more confidence. Gaining confidence was important to me, since I was chubby as a little girl. As I got into my teen years, I strived to be in shape.

When I started college at the University of Wisconsin-Madison, I began teaching fitness classes three days a week at the athletic center on campus. I enjoyed every minute of it and taught classes throughout my four years in college. It was not only fun to teach packed classes of 250 students at a time, which included many of my sorority sisters, business school classmates, and other friends, but it was also a great way to ward off stress while carrying a busy class load, taking exams, and participating in many extracurricular activities and social events. In addition, teaching gave me solid public speaking experience and the ability to help others lead a healthy lifestyle during college.

After graduating college and starting my corporate career, I continued to teach fitness and dance classes on the side and decided to train, in my free time, for an ESPN fitness competition. I first saw the competition on TV when I was in college and thought it was an amazing and unique blend of fitness, dance, and gymnastics, which was right up my alley. I worked with a trainer, coach, and choreographer and trained six days per week for two to three hours a day for months on end over the course of three years.

It was hard work, and doing the training sessions early in the mornings before work or late in the evenings after a long day of work was grueling. However, it was worth it to me since I enjoyed the rewards of training and the thrill of competing. I was extremely committed and determined to do well in the competition, as my goal was to place in the top three.

In my first year competing, I placed ninth in the West Coast regionals in San Francisco, which was a good start. In my second year, I competed in Los Angeles and placed first and qualified for the national competition in Miami. When training for and competing at nationals, I worked hard; overcame injuries, obstacles, and fears; channeled my inner passions and spirit, and fortunately placed second and took home the silver medal. I also had a brief appearance on ESPN, which made my younger self so happy after all those years of doing workout shows on ESPN and training so hard for this competition.

In addition to dance and fitness, I've also enjoyed running with my husband over the years. We've trained for and run a marathon, half marathon, and several 5K and 10K races together. We're both very goal-oriented and active, and training for races or events has always been a challenging and fun outlet for us as individuals and as a couple.

When I was pregnant with each of my sons, I continued to make exercise and movement an integral part of my life because I knew it would make me stronger throughout my pregnancy and when going through labor. I did a lot of walking, prenatal yoga, Pilates, and strength training with light hand weights. As my body changed during pregnancy and caused aches and pains, exercise is what saved me. It helped to reduce the pain and allowed me to feel more like my normal self by staying active. I also was able to quickly get back to my fitness regimen once I received the green light from my doctor six weeks postpartum. I bounced back and recovered more easily since I had exercised throughout both of my pregnancies.

As you can see from my experiences, I kept moving, literally and figuratively, through various stages of my life. Movement was so helpful in keeping me mentally and physically strong throughout childhood, middle school, high school, college, graduate school, my career, pregnancy, and motherhood. However, when my life got busier as a working mom and I stopped exercising and dancing regularly, I really saw a difference in myself. I lacked energy and motivation, and my mood often shifted. As a result, I didn't feel very happy and fulfilled and, instead, felt cranky and defeated. I wasn't as strong and felt physically and emotionally weak. My confidence suffered, and I truly lost a vital piece of myself.

Realizing what I had given up and the negative impact it was having on me is what pushed me to make a change. I yearned for transformation and wanted to get back that piece of myself that I'd lost. So I put one foot in front of the other and slowly started exercising and dancing more. I eventually found my way back to movement and wellness, and for that, I'll always be truly grateful.

Where does movement fit into your life? Have you had periods when it played a smaller or bigger role or no role at all? It's possible to make movement a regular part of your life if it isn't already. Here are four ways to get started or to continue to do it, even if there are times when you get stuck.

1. Pick activities you enjoy.

Do you enjoy doing boot camps, interval training, strength training, dance, Pilates, yoga, running, walking, cycling, sports, or other outdoor activities? Since everyone has different interests and abilities, find what makes you tick and tap into that. If you enjoy what you're doing, you're more likely to stick with it and make it a habit. Instead of dreading exercise, you'll be able to look forward to it and know it can be a lifelong tool to help you through various aspects of your life. I have clients who like dance above any other type of workout, so they tend to only take my dance classes and make the most out of them. I have other clients who like my low-intensity Pilates, yoga, and sculpt classes due to knee or back injuries and don't have an interest in dance or high-intensity classes. They know their interest and ability levels and exercise within those parameters.

That said, have a variety of activities you enjoy and participate in so you don't get bored or hit a plateau from a fitness perspective. Even if you love a certain activity, doing the same thing all the time can get old, and you also risk getting overuse injuries, which can occur when you're using the same muscles and doing the same movements over and over again. Pick a few different activities you can rotate and do on different days and weeks so you can cross-train, enjoy your workouts, stay challenged, and prevent injuries.

2. Find a community or a workout buddy.

Do you have an in-person or online fitness community you're a part of? Having accountability partners is critical to sticking with a fitness regimen and ensuring movement is a consistent part of your day-to-day life. Whether you work out with your spouse or significant other, sister, girlfriends, fellow attendees in classes at the gym or park, an online community, or other group, find people in your life who can hold you accountable and who you can hold accountable. Having this support system of people who want to see one another succeed will be invaluable, especially on those days when you're feeling unmotivated or lacking confidence.

I recently had a discussion with a few of my regular students who take my in-person and livestream fitness classes. They talked about how helpful it is to have a group of people you know are going to be in class regularly. It especially helps on those days when it's hard to get out of bed early or get in the right mindset to exercise. If others show up, then it's easier to also show up for them and yourself. Also, having an instructor who believes in you, sees the best in you, and can encourage and push you, especially when you can't do it for yourself, is extremely beneficial. These are some of the many reasons why I fell in love with group fitness all those years ago as a college student, and why I continue to teach group fitness and build communities year after year.

3. Find times of the day that are most realistic for you to exercise.

When it comes to determining when to exercise each day, be honest with yourself about the blocks of time that will be most realistic for you. Are you a morning person? Do you prefer to exercise during lunchtime to break up the day? Are evenings a good time to exercise and decompress after a long day of work? Pay attention to your natural rhythms, schedule, and lifestyle preferences, and prioritize exercise accordingly.

I personally prefer to work out in the morning. It sets a positive tone for the day, allows me to infuse my mind and body with energy and strength, and it's done early, so I can focus on my family, work, and other tasks throughout the rest of the day. However, I'm not one to exercise as early as 6:00 a.m. For me, the ideal time is 9:00 a.m., after getting dressed, making breakfast for my family, getting my kids organized and off to school, and before I shower and start my workday.

My clients have varying preferences for when to exercise, and they're usually based on the type of job they have, the age of their kids, the types of exercise they prefer, and what resources and equipment they have access to at home or outside their home. I always tell them that something is better than nothing, and constant and consistent movement day-to-day and week-to-week can really add up!

4. Use a wearable device.

In my opinion, wearable devices such as a Fitbit or Apple watch are like mini wellness coaches on your wrist that travel with you throughout the day. They remind you of how many steps you've taken, how many calories you've burned, when you should stand up and move if you've been sitting for too long, when to take deep breaths to practice mindfulness, how many hours of sleep you're getting, and so much more. Wearable devices provide data—data translates into knowledge, and knowledge is power. You're in the driver's seat when it comes to your lifestyle choices, and having access to information can empower you to make the best choices you can for your health and well-being every day. The key is to not get obsessive about the data or let it run your life. Consider the data points and then make informed decisions that are right for you, your mind, and your body, and allow you to still enjoy your life. This insight is based on my own experiences using a Fitbit and my clients' experiences using their own wearable devices as they work to achieve their goals.

5. Leverage technology.

Living and working in Silicon Valley for many years has taught me a lot about technology. It certainly leads to innovation and has the ability to make life more efficient, connected, and accessible. At the same time, it can create stress and anxiety, make us feel like we're always on, and be difficult to disconnect from on a daily basis.

However, I want to focus on how technology can be used for good, as I like to say. When we're using our smartphones, wearable devices, and social media channels for the purposes of doing workouts, listening to guided meditations, and connecting with others within an online community, we're using technology in a productive way.

I want to encourage you to use online health and fitness videos, apps, livestream classes, courses, and live virtual events as helpful tools to get in your workouts. They can complement other activities you might participate in, such as classes at the gym or outside, running, walking, hiking, and playing sports. I recommend apps such as MyFitnessPal and Strava, online videos such as Daily Burn, Beachbody, POPSUGAR Fitness, my Passion Fit YouTube channel, and my live Passion Fit virtual events through Facebook and Instagram. After you've used technology for good, as well as for work and entertainment, I suggest you put it away so you can live and enjoy your life to the fullest with the ones you love.

QUESTIONS

1. How can exercise and movement help you, beyond just physically?

2. What time of the day would be most realistic to get your workouts done?

3. What dance, fitness, or sport activities do you enjoy most?

4. Are you able to invest in a wearable device to take your progress to the next level?

5. What can you do to get movement back into your life if you fall off-track or get stuck, and who can be your accountability partners to help you if that happens?

CHAPTER 7

SLEEP ON IT ... TOMORROW WILL BE A NEW DAY

IT'S THE MIDDLE OF THE NIGHT, and you either get up to go to the bathroom or grab a glass of water. Or maybe you wake up because your spouse or significant other is snoring or your kids come into your room after a bad dream and need reassurance to go back to bed. Or maybe you simply need to change sleep positions. Before you know it, you're wide awake and can't fall back asleep. Ugh! Has this ever happened to you, and if so, don't you hate when it happens?! This has definitely happened to me, where something external causes me to wake up and then I find myself wide awake. But at other times, I can't sleep because of other reasons.

For instance, I always know that when something is

weighing on me or when I've been working too much or spending too much time on screens—especially close to bedtime—it will severely affect my sleep. Luckily, I don't usually have problems falling asleep, but I can have a tendency to wake up in the middle of the night with my mind racing, and it becomes difficult to fall back asleep. If you've ever had this experience, you may have symptoms of insomnia.

I've experienced insomnia during different stages in my life: when my kids were newborns, when I worked crazy hours, when I contemplated changing careers, and when I worried about close family members who were dealing with health issues. Over the last few years, I've made a conscious effort to better manage my sleep by practicing what industry experts often call good sleep-hygiene techniques, which I share with you later in this chapter.

I've learned through my experiences that sleep is one of the most essential aspects of good health and the ability to be a high-functioning human being. Its importance can't be underestimated, and the best way to realize that is to pay attention to how you feel when you get a good night's sleep compared to when you don't. You're likely to feel energetic, alert, and able to think clearly and be in a good mood when you've slept well. When you haven't slept well, you might feel lethargic, unmotivated, exhausted, and in a bad mood.

It's critical to protect your sleep at all costs. No matter what might be happening in your life, at the end of the day, it's time to sleep on it and remember that tomorrow will be a new day. According to the Centers for Disease Control and Prevention, adults who get less than seven hours of sleep per night are more likely to develop chronic health conditions, such as asthma, coronary heart disease, and arthritis, compared to those who get the recommended amount of seven to nine hours. A lack of sleep can also impact your memory, alertness, other cognitive abilities, relationships, career, and more, because you won't be able to operate at full capacity or function at your best.

Sometimes our sleep may be disrupted by situations outside of our control, and at other times, it may be related to something internal. Instead of just chalking it up to the fact that you're a light sleeper, dig deep and figure out what's happening in your life that may be causing you stress or worry, either consciously or unconsciously. Are you or your spouse or significant other facing pressures at work? Are you worried about your kids? Is anyone in your family dealing with any health issues? Are you dealing with any health issues? Is something about the future making you uneasy?

It may not always be a fun process to dig into some of your deepest fears or issues occurring in your life, but it's a necessary step to help you get to the bottom of what's impacting your sleep. It may help to talk to family, close friends, or a professional. Also, you may want to get in touch with your doctor if the issue continues to persist and impacts your day-to-day life or your health.

Getting the right quantity, quality, and consistency of sleep is important for your overall health. Below are some of the many health benefits of a good night's sleep, according to an article written by Joe Leech, MS, and medically reviewed by Atli Arnarson, BSc, PhD, in *healthline*:

- Reduces risk of weight gain
- Improves concentration
- Increases productivity
- Strengthens athletic performance
- Decreases risk of heart attack
- Decreases risk of stroke
- Decreases risk of diabetes
- Keeps metabolism in control
- Improves immune system
- Reduces risk of depression and anxiety
- Reduces inflammation
- Improves social and emotional health

Oftentimes, we take our sleep for granted, but it is essential to prioritize our need for sleep throughout our life, especially before more serious issues arise. If you want to reap these benefits and prevent future health issues, try one or more of the following sleep-hygiene techniques.

Create the right sleep environment.

Is your bedroom set up in such a way that promotes healthy sleep, or could there be elements in your room that may be hindering it? Believe it or not, the aesthetics of your bedroom can make a big difference. Having calming and warm paint colors on the walls, such as light blue, light green, violet, pastel pink, pale yellow, or tan, could work well. Sleeping with soft and comfortable sheets, comforters, and pillows also help to ensure you feel cozy at night.

Room temperature impacts your sleep environment, and

you may need to negotiate it with your spouse or significant other. My husband and I usually have nightly debates over this because he's always hot and I'm always cold. However, you don't want the room to be too hot or too cold. Ideally, medical experts suggest a temperature between 65 and 72 degrees for optimal sleep.

Finally, sound and light also affect your sleep environment. Ensure you have window treatments that block out light, especially early in the morning. Also, whether you live in the city, the suburbs, or the country, and whether your environment is loud or quiet, having a noise-canceling sound machine or ear plugs could help. Some people are more sensitive to sound and light than others, so do what's best for your sleep, and don't be afraid to test out different options if needed.

Manage technology.

Technology is another element of sleep to be considered. Usually, most people have different needs, opinions, and choices on this one. One of the first considerations is whether or not to have a TV in your bedroom. Some people are against it, and others enjoy having one. My husband and I do have a TV in our bedroom, but we try to ensure we turn it off and leave enough time to wind down before going to sleep. For us, it's worth it because we often like to relax and watch a movie upstairs in the evenings or in the mornings on the weekends with the kids. What's important is to create boundaries with the TV and ensure it's not on all the time or negatively impacting your sleep.

Other screens, such as laptops, tablets, and smartphones, can also affect your sleep. It's pretty common for many people to work on their laptops, watch a Netflix show on their tablets, or scroll through social media on their smartphones in bed at night. Let's face it—we all do this from time to time, and maybe some people do it more frequently than others. However, boundaries are needed here too. Set a time when screens are shut down so your brain doesn't get overstimulated—ideally thirty to sixty minutes before bedtime. And if you have children—the same rules would apply to them.

One thing that's helped me over the last year is charging my smartphone outside my and my husband's bedroom. I charge it near an outlet in the hallway, so I can still hear my alarm in the morning, but the smartphone isn't sitting on my nightstand with the distracting blue light, the notification bells ringing, and the sheer temptation to check email or social media when I should be reading, practicing mindfulness, journaling, or simply winding down. It has made a huge difference for me, and I've recommended it to a few of my clients. Feel free to try it too!

Deal with negative thoughts.

Another culprit of a poor night's sleep is when you can't get negative thoughts out of your mind. I'm not going to lie; this one can be tough. However, having go-to strategies can help. One strategy is to acknowledge your thoughts but then tell yourself you're going to shift your mindset to a different and positive thought instead. For example, if your negative thought is that your new boss at work may be tough to work with, perhaps you can shift your thinking and tell yourself you'll keep an open mind, look for positive qualities, and make the best of the working relationship. Another strategy is to write down the negative thought on a Post-it note (for example, *I feel like I'm never going to lose the weight I put on during pregnancy*) and then crumple it up and throw it away. This can be both empowering and liberating if you do it consistently. A third strategy is to practice mindfulness by taking deep breaths and only focusing on your breathing to get the stressful thoughts out of your mind. Other aspects of mindfulness could include praying or listening to calming music to change your mental state.

Write down what's keeping you awake.

If you're unable to sleep because of general stress, a difficult conversation you had that day, or forgetting something you have to do the next day, writing down what's keeping you awake can help you release those thoughts from your mind. By doing so, you acknowledge the thoughts and then give yourself permission to deal with them in the future, which allows you to carry on with your night's sleep. It also helps to keep a notebook and pen on your nightstand so you can instantly write out your thoughts or even make a list of what you have to get done, if those bothersome thoughts wake you up during the night. Trust me, you'll feel so much better when you take all of those thoughts that swirl around in your mind and put them down on paper. You'll feel good knowing you've captured everything and have a plan for dealing with them the next day.

Keep a consistent sleep schedule.

While life is often busy and unpredictable, stay consistent with your sleep schedule as much as possible so you can handle all that may come your way. While it's not always easy to do so if you travel frequently (especially to different time zones) or socialize a lot on the weekends, the more you can wake up and go to sleep at the same time, the more you're training your mind and body to follow suit. You'll also have a better chance of getting the recommended seven to nine hours of sleep per night and perhaps even more than that.

I remember how hard my husband and I tried to have a consistent sleeping and napping schedule for our kids, especially when they were babies and toddlers. We did that for a reason: to ensure they were developing and functioning properly. As adults, it's important we do that for ourselves.

We owe it to ourselves, our families, our friends, and our employers to give the best version of us in each situation. Consistent sleep is what will allow us to be rested, calm, clearheaded, rational, kind, and productive. If you want to feel successful in your personal and professional life, and maintain good health, remember that sleep is one of your greatest assets!

QUESTIONS

1. How many hours of sleep are you currently getting per night?

2. Do you have the right environment for sleep in your bedroom?

3. Do stressful thoughts, worries, or your to-do lists keep you up at night? Are there certain stressors in your life that negatively impact your sleep? If so, which sleep-hygiene techniques might work best for you?

4. Can you rethink how you use screens at night in your bedroom and what changes you can make so that technology and your devices don't hinder your sleep? What adjustments might you make?

5. What might a consistent sleep schedule look like for you based on your career, family, and lifestyle?

CHAPTER 8

EXPECT THE UNEXPECTED AND GET READY TO FIRE ON ALL CYLINDERS!

PRODUCTIVITY IS CRITICAL to accomplishing tasks, reaching goals, and being successful, whether as an individual, as part of an organization, or within your own business. In my opinion, in order to be more productive, it's crucial to first manage your health and well-being. When you're healthy, you're able to truly engage in your work and personal life. That, in turn, allows you to be more productive and ultimately more successful.

According to a Gallup research study mentioned in a January 16, 2019, article written by Naz Beheshti in *Forbes*, entitled "10 Timely Statistics About the Connection Between Employee Engagement and Wellness," highly engaged teams show 21 percent more profitability. This finding makes a lot of sense because when you're more engaged and producing more, you'll inevitably be able to achieve positive results, including increased profits. And in this study and article, engagement is defined as showing up each day with passion, purpose, presence, and energy. I believe these attributes are heavily tied to your mindset, health, and well-being.

Many of my clients are busy moms who are also juggling demanding careers and/or volunteer work. They're physicians, nurses, lawyers, engineers, environmentalists, entrepreneurs, teachers, principals, pharmacists, marketers, tech execs, and PTA leaders. Although their duties and responsibilities vary, one thing they often share with me is that being able to focus on their mental and physical health helps them stay engaged, productive, and on track. Over time, they've come to realize that if they can prioritize something as simple as waking up refreshed after a good night's sleep, a quick workout to get their bodies moving, or a few minutes of mindfulness to get centered, they're able to set the tone for the day and accomplish great things.

Now, even with the best of intentions to set the tone for an engaged and productive day, unexpected challenges can pop up. If you're a mama with young children and you work from home, you especially know what I'm talking about. Or if you're juggling work in an office or another workplace facility with school-aged kids who require school drop-offs and pick-ups, forgotten homework assignments, lunchboxes, and more, you probably can relate. And whether or not you have kids, other unexpected occurrences such as traffic jams, client issues, and new projects can also throw off your productivity.

I have a funny story about how my productivity and the flow of my morning were completely thrown off several years ago. It wasn't funny at the time, but at least I can laugh about it and share the story with you now. My husband was out of town, traveling for work, and I was solo with our two boys and busy with work, which had become a common scenario at that time. Our older son was five years old and in kindergarten, and our younger son was two years old and in preschool. On this particular morning, I had a big presentation to give at work for several executive clients who were flying in from out of town.

I knew I had a lot on my plate; however, I initially felt like I was firing on all cylinders. I was well prepared for my presentation, got up early so I could shower and get myself ready, with ample time left to get my kids dressed, fed, and ready for school. Everything was going according to plan, and I was even operating ahead of schedule ... or so I thought. Unfortunately, soon after, my older son came into the bathroom while I was putting on my makeup and said, "Mommy, come with me. You *have* to see this!" I nervously said okay, and he grabbed my hand and led me to the hallway.

When I saw the sight in front of me, I didn't know whether to cry or shriek in shock and horror. My younger son, who we were starting to potty train, didn't tell me he had to go to the bathroom and didn't make it in time by himself. He was running around without his pants or Pull-Ups and had proceeded to go number two all over the carpet in the hallway and somehow had managed to smear it all over himself and several toys in his room. He said, "I sorry, Mommy." I couldn't believe it. I told him it was okay but thought to myself, *Is this really happening?!* I was frozen in panic, but then I looked at my watch and realized if I didn't move fast, I would be late dropping off the kids to school and getting to my work meeting.

I scrambled and started running a bath, picked up my younger son, and put him in the bathtub. As I was giving him a quick bath, I tried my best to hold it together, but tears started to run down my cheeks. My older son, who felt bad for me, began to rub my back and said, "It's okay, Mommy. It's okay." It was impossible not to notice how sweet and helpful he was acting and how my little one was trying his best to be helpful too.

After finishing up the bath and getting my younger son dressed again, I grabbed a big stack of baby wipes, picked up the mess on the carpet, and threw it all in the Diaper Genie. I then washed all the toys with soap and hot water, sprayed the carpet with carpet cleaner, and tried to get the stains out with a sponge. That was the best I could do in the moment, and I figured I would do a deeper cleaning in the evening after work. After that, I washed my hands thoroughly!

Once the kids and I were ready to go, I realized I no longer had enough time to drop off both kids and make it to work on time. I asked one of my best friends and neighbors if she could take my five-year-old to school with her son who was the same age so I only had to drive my younger son to preschool before I drove to the office.

I made it to work in the nick of time, and when a few of my fellow working mom friends saw me, they asked if I was ready for my big presentation. I looked at them, and my eyes started to fill up with tears again. I felt like a mess and told them about my morning. Because they could completely understand and relate to what had happened, they immediately gave me huge hugs and shared their own similar stories with me. They gave me a quick pep talk, told me I would still do well in my presentation, and encouraged me to get out there and do my best. I was so incredibly thankful for them in that moment and still to this day. Working moms are a force! They gave me the gift of empathy and confidence, which gave me the strength I needed to nail my presentation.

The moral of this story is: You never know what's going to happen each day. Distractions, chaos, and many other unexpected events will undoubtedly occur. However, to stay productive and engaged, you have to expect the unexpected, deal with it (and help from friends, family, neighbors, and co-workers is always a blessing), and then keep on going. Don't let the chaos completely throw you off course. I know it's easier said than done, but if you stay strong and continue to move forward, before you know it, you'll be firing on all cylinders once again!

Additionally, it helps to have solid productivity tools to rely on so you can keep moving forward with your day, even if unexpected events occur. Here are five of my favorites you can apply to your personal and professional life.

1. Make "top three" personal and professional to-do lists.

While it's common for people to make to-do lists, it took me years to figure out that streamlining them is a critical step for success. Throughout college and graduate school, I made long, ambitious, and often unattainable to-do lists, which basically set me up for failure. Early on in my career, after reading a number of books on time management and productivity and getting helpful feedback from my managers and career mentors, I finally realized the power and liberation that came from focusing primarily on my top three personal and professional tasks to get done each day. These could be written down in a notebook (which is what I prefer) or entered into an online tool or app such as Wunderlist, Todoist, or Trello.

From a work perspective, they needed to be strategic, mission-critical, revenue-generating, and needle-moving tasks. From a personal perspective, they needed to be the most pressing, long-term-driven, or life-enriching tasks. Before moving on to anything else, these tasks would need to be completed, and if they were, I felt successful. If I was able to tackle more on my to-do list, that was great. But if not, I knew I still would be accomplishing a great deal to make my day impactful.

2. Have an organized work space and calendar.

It's no secret that organization is another key to productivity and success. While we all have our own styles and preferences, figure out what types of organizational tactics work best for you. As I've mentioned before, I'm a Type A personality, so if I'm not organized, I get stressed out. To stay organized, I try to make sure I create folders and subfolders for my emails, electronic and paper files, and documents.

I also try to ensure my work space is clear with just my computer, phone, a notebook, pen, and any paperwork I may be reviewing. I try not to have a ton of clutter around me, and if I have a pile of mail, books, documents, or anything else I need to review, I try to keep the piles neat and orderly so they, once again, don't stress me out. It helps me keep my head clear and my mind focused on the task at hand.

In addition, as mentioned earlier, my calendar is another great organizational tool. I use Google Calendar (of course!) and color code my meetings, appointments, deadlines, travel, volunteer work, social plans, relaxation, and anything that doesn't fall into one of these main categories. I also have different colors for anything on my calendar that pertains to my kids or husband. Now, this might be too much organization for you, but again, the key is to find a system that works for you and then stick with it and develop consistency. It will allow you to prepare and run your day versus having your day run you.

3. Stay laser-focused, but take breaks.

When it comes to work, I can get laser-focused and stay in the zone for hours on end. But over time, I've learned from my own mistakes and experiences that it's essential to take breaks in order to produce your best work.

Several years ago, I took a course developed by The Energy Project called "Managing Your Energy and Not Your Time," and in that course, they talked about the importance of taking breaks every ninety minutes. When you do this, you'll have a chance to get up and move, grab a glass of water, make a phone call, talk to a co-worker, go outdoors and soak up some sunshine, or whatever else you may need to do. You can clear your mind so you can reenergize and refocus once the break is over. You'll be able to produce more high-quality work than you would if you had kept powering through your workday without taking a break. My husband is really good at doing this, and he's one of the most productive people I know. Seriously, he's a machine! So take it from me (and my husband), and take those breaks every ninety minutes to continue operating like the superstar you are!

4. Get in movement throughout the workday.

Another key aspect of productivity, which goes along with taking breaks, is to get movement in throughout your workday. While it might sound counterintuitive or like a distraction, it's important for not only your work, but your overall health and well-being. When you're sitting and working at a computer for long hours at a time, you're being sedentary. It's no better than sitting on a couch and watching TV for long hours at a time. The impact on your body, metabolism, blood sugar, blood flow, and more is the same. As medical experts often say these days, sitting is the new smoking. Make the time to move by taking a walk outside for ten minutes, doing some stretches at your desk, scheduling a workout at lunchtime, using a standing desk, sitting on a Swiss ball instead of a regular chair, or any other activity that allows you to move your body on a regular basis throughout your workday. Trust me, it will do wonders for your work performance and health!

5. Set up a reward system.

With all this discussion about productivity, it's also important to take a moment to appreciate what you accomplish. Just like we often set up reward systems for our kids for good behavior, finishing their homework, or eating their vegetables, who's to say adults can't enjoy some rewards too? Now maybe M&M's or sticker rewards aren't your thing, but you can pick whatever rewards (big or small) would be most motivating for you.

For example, if you complete a big project at work by the deadline at the end of the month, then perhaps you can buy a new outfit or a pair of shoes. Or if you're able to learn to cook two new healthy recipes this week, then you might treat yourself and your family to some frozen yogurt at the end of the week. You get the idea. Get creative and come up with rewards that will encourage you to be focused and productive and reach your goals.

Finally, try to apply a growth mindset toward productivity. If you stay focused on the process of learning and growing along the way versus stressing yourself out about the outcome, you're more likely to feel fulfilled by completing your goals and to feel deserving of your rewards. So make your top three to-do lists, get organized, be focused, but take breaks, keep moving, set up your reward system, and enjoy the journey!

QUESTIONS

1. Do you like to write out your to-do lists or enter them into an online tool or app?

2. What type of organizational and calendar system would work best for you and be most realistic to keep up with?

3. How can you remind yourself to take breaks every ninety minutes during your workday? Enter them into your calendar? Set a timer? Use your wearable device? Something else?

4. How can you keep moving your body throughout your day to avoid being sedentary at your desk and computer?

5. What rewards would be most motivating for you to reach your personal and professional goals?

CHAPTER 9

HEY HONEY, WHAT'S FOR DINNER?

"HEY HONEY, WHAT'S FOR DINNER?" I'm sure for many of you, this is a question you either ask or get asked by your significant other often, if not daily. And if you have kids, they're probably asking the same thing. My family and I are in the same boat! While this question represents yet one more task we have to get done each day, it's one for us all to carefully consider, whether it's dinner or any other meal that's being discussed.

Nutrition plays such a key role in how we feel and function and has a huge impact on our brains, bodies, overall health, and well-being, both now and in the future as we age. But when we're busy, tired, and short on time, we often take shortcuts and end up making choices that are less than stellar for our health. Let's face it, we've all been there, and it's completely understandable!

That said, based on my training and certification as a nutrition specialist, I want to share some nutrition philosophies and tips that have worked well for my family and me and can be tweaked and changed as needed. Although there is specific information that everyone can look to for guidance, nutrition needs to be personalized for each individual. We all have different body types, genetic predispositions, taste preferences, potential food allergies, or other dietary restrictions that require consideration. However, I'm hoping these insights will allow you to view nutrition and healthy eating in a new and fresh way without feeling like you have to be a slave to every new diet trend out there or spend hours in the kitchen. Variety, balance, and simplicity are key, and there are ways to properly fuel your body to increase your performance in all areas of your life and still enjoy your food. In this chapter, we'll take a look at how to do this.

According to the President's Council on Sports, Fitness & Nutrition, typical diets in the US far exceed the recommended levels of sugars, fats, refined grains, and sodium. This information is troublesome because regularly eating these types of foods can lead to obesity and other potential health issues, such as diabetes. Pay close attention to what you're putting in your body so you can not only prevent long-term health issues and diseases, but you can also optimize your health, career, and life as a wellness-empowered woman.

Now, I know it sometimes can be confusing to determine what's best to put in your body because there are always new diet trends taking shape, ongoing research on nutrition, and ever-changing food guidelines. For these reasons, my philosophies on nutrition focus on the traditional Mediterranean style of eating, which includes tried-and-true food principles that have been around for decades and allow for clean eating, balance, and moderation.

My mom has had a big influence on my nutritional philosophies because her approach has always been natural and sensible. For instance, she focuses on whole foods versus processed foods and the enjoyment of all foods in moderation versus depriving yourself. I've seen, firsthand, how effective this approach can be. My approach has also been influenced by my ongoing training and education in nutrition and observing what has worked for my clients and me.

Also, being a part of the dance and fitness world for most of my life, I've unfortunately witnessed many people with eating disorders and unhealthy views on food. While I've always been conscious of what I eat, I've wanted to be a good role model for healthy eating and maintaining a safe and healthy relationship with food. In fact, while in college, I often publicly spoke about the dangers of eating disorders to all of the students who took my fitness classes, and I offered resources on campus if anyone was struggling. Unfortunately, eating disorders were and continue to be a common occurrence for many young women in college and at other stages of life as well. My goal now is to continue to educate women of all ages and provide mindsets and tools around food and nutrition to help them make healthy and informed choices that have as much to do with their mental health as they do with their physical health.

Here are my thoughts on the foundations of a healthy eating plan based on the latest research. Some of this information may already be familiar to you, and some of it may be new. Either way, it's summarized here for you as a reminder or reference point, and to give you healthy meal ideas, since nutrition is such an integral part of holistic wellness. It will allow you to function at your best, both personally and professionally.

Fruits and vegetables: Let's start with a major part of any nutrition plan, which includes organic and plant-based foods, such as fruits and vegetables. These foods are natural, grown from the ground up, and are filled with vitamins, minerals, and nutrients. Federal guidelines recommend getting one to two cups of fruit and two to three cups of vegetables per day, depending on how many total calories you're consuming each day. Incorporating colorful fruits and vegetables, such as broccoli, kale, spinach, tomatoes, zucchini, apples, oranges, bananas, blueberries, and grapes, can provide you with vitamins A, C, E, folic acid, fiber, potassium, magnesium, iron, antioxidants, flavonoids, and calcium to protect against various diseases and keep your body functioning well.

Fruits and vegetables can be eaten as standalone snacks or can be paired with other foods and baked, sautéed, or grilled as part of a larger meal. Add them to healthy baked breads, protein dishes, salads, soups, stews, oatmeal, smoothies, sandwiches, and more. The key is to eat a variety of fruits and vegetables in order to maximize your nutritional intake, make your meals more interesting and colorful, and prevent you and your family from getting bored with eating the same meals over and over. You can also buy a combo of fresh and frozen fruits and vegetables at the grocery store so you have more options over an extended period.

Protein: Getting an adequate amount of protein every day is critical for creating lean muscle mass in the body, giving you energy by carrying oxygen in your blood, and building and repairing tissues, cells, bones, skin, and cartilage. Whether you're vegetarian, vegan, or a meat-eater, there are many options for getting protein in your meals. Some examples of proteins across all of these categories include beans, lentils, tofu, chicken, fish, turkey, pork, and eggs.

No matter what types of protein you include in your nutrition plan, I recommend that you shop organic and natural, whenever possible, versus purchasing processed foods. This ensures increased nutrients and decreased chemicals. Also, pay attention to the levels of saturated fats, trans fats, cholesterol, and sodium to ensure they're not too high or present at all. In addition, I encourage you to buy and cook your protein dishes in bulk at the beginning of each week so you can easily create multiple meals with less cooking time during the week. For example, beans can be used in salads, burritos, and dips with healthy, whole-grain crackers or chips. Ground turkey meat can be used in whole-grain pasta dishes as well as chili dishes, lettuce wraps, or stir-fries. If you get creative and plan your meals ahead of time, you can build around the protein dishes and figure out what side dishes, including vegetables, to include to maximize efficiency and variety.

Whole grains: A lot of debate has taken place over the years around carbohydrates, refined grains, and whole grains.

We've also been introduced to many low-carb styles of eating, such as the Keto and Paleo diets, which many people do for weight loss, food allergies, or other health concerns. For these reasons, there isn't a one-size-fits-all approach to nutrition because everyone does have such unique needs. That being said, be sure to include foods from all the major food groups into your meals, if at all possible, because the human body needs most or all of the nutrients that come from these foods to function optimally and fight diseases.

When it comes to carbohydrates and grains, the key is to focus on complex carbohydrates and whole grains versus simple carbohydrates and refined grains. Instead of eating white bread, pasta, and rice, your meals would ideally include whole-grain bread, oatmeal, and pasta; brown rice, quinoa, barley, couscous, and the like. If you have any dietary restrictions or gluten allergies, you can choose gluten-free options.

These grains should be eaten in moderation. For example, if you're having oatmeal and fruit for breakfast and a sandwich for lunch, it's probably best not to eat grains with dinner. Instead, focus on getting protein and vegetables in that meal to moderate your grain intake for the day. The key ideas here are balance and the quality of grains!

Healthy fats: Many misconceptions and debates exist when it comes to fats. We do need to avoid or seriously minimize cholesterol, saturated, and trans fats found in foods such as potato chips, French fries, cookies, and cakes. However, monounsaturated and polyunsaturated fats found in foods such as olive oil, avocados, nuts, seeds, and fish are the healthy fats we need. These types of healthy fats are packed with vitamins, minerals, and nutrients and have many benefits.

Healthy fats can protect against heart disease, cancer, and diabetes. They can increase the development and function of your brain. They can protect your body from cellular damage. They can reduce inflammation. They can make you feel full and slow down your digestion. They can decrease blood pressure and so much more. I encourage you to be mindful of the composition of fats you cook with and put into your body so you can minimize the bad ones and maximize the good ones. Paying close attention to your fat intake is one of the most beneficial things you can do to protect your health and longevity.

Low-fat dairy: Dairy is one more food group that works for some people and not for others, and in recent years, it seems to have received a negative reputation. If you're lactose intolerant, you'll obviously need to check with your doctor about which dairy foods to avoid and to learn about lactose-free alternatives. However, there are many health benefits to eating dairy foods such as milk, yogurt, and cheese, as long as you eat them in moderation, pay attention to the amount of cholesterol, sugar, and saturated and trans fats in them, and opt for low-fat versions. Low-fat dairy foods provide calcium, vitamin D, vitamin B, and protein, and are good for bone health and gut health.

For women, it's also important to get enough calcium and vitamin D to protect against osteoporosis, and if it's not possible to get them from low-fat dairy foods, you can talk to your doctor about supplements or even dairy-free substitutes that still contain calcium and vitamin D, such as almond milk.

Regardless of your stance on dairy, focus on what works for you and ensure you're getting the nutrients needed from dairy foods or their healthy substitutes to maximize your health and well-being.

Water: In addition to eating healthy foods to optimize your health and performance both personally and professionally, hydrating your body with water is equally critical. According to an article that was medically reviewed by Jillian Kubala, MS, RD, and written by Claire Sissons in *Medical News Today*, about 60 percent of the human body is made up of water. Dehydration at varying degrees can lead to health issues such as headaches, lethargy, water retention, bloating, constipation, and more serious issues such as kidney problems, urinary problems, a decrease in blood supply, shock, or even seizures.

Have you heard the traditional advice to drink eight, eight-ounce glasses of water each day? While that's a great general guideline, people are different shapes, sizes, and weights, and we need some level of customization. The rule of thumb I always share with my clients is to drink half your body weight in ounces of water. For example, if you weigh 120 pounds, you'll want to aim to consume sixty ounces of water each day. And if you're in hot, humid weather or exercising, you'll want to consume more. Also, be sure to replace electrolytes that are lost when your body is subjected to extreme heat or vigorous workouts. Adding a low-sugar supplement or powder to your water is important in those situations.

While it can be challenging to make the time to cook and eat healthy meals with your family, it's definitely worth it.

And if you're a mom, by doing so, you'll be a good role model for your kids and can set a positive example of what healthy eating looks like. Nutrition is critical for being at your best in your personal and professional life and for protecting and optimizing your health. And using apps like MyFitnessPal can help you easily track your meals, analyze the nutrition content and portion sizes of the food you're cooking and eating, and provide you with an overall awareness of your food intake. Remember, variety, balance, and simplicity are key. With a little planning, preparation, and commitment, it's possible to easily make meals that contain these delicious foods. So what are you waiting for? Get creative and get cooking! You can do it!

QUESTIONS

1. What's your biggest challenge when it comes to preparing healthy meals?

2. What's one thing you can start doing to prioritize healthy eating?

3. What are some of your and your family's favorite fruits, vegetables, proteins, and grains that you can start with and then build more meal ideas from there?

4. How can you simplify your meal planning, grocery shopping, and cooking processes?

5. Did you learn any new information about nutrition that you can take note of and incorporate into your meal planning, or was this information more of a reminder for you?

CHAPTER 10

WHO LOVES YOU, BABY?

I OFTEN TALK ABOUT WHAT I CALL "The 3 Fs," which stand for family, friends, and fun. In my opinion, "The 3 Fs" are what life is all about. We all need to work hard and pursue our goals, passions, and dreams, but if we're not able to spend enough time with our family and friends and to have fun in life, what's it all for anyway?

While this philosophy might seem obvious, it's amazing how often people lose sight of it, myself included—especially while smack in the middle of a global pandemic, which completely turned our world upside down, and for most of us, made it even more challenging. However, while in quarantine in California with my family during the COVID-19 shutdown, I can tell you it made me reevaluate my life priorities and helped me see my eternal gratitude for my family and friends. For these reasons, I want to spend time discussing this significant life topic. I'd like to share my personal insights, based on my own experiences with prioritizing (and not prioritizing) "The 3 Fs" in various stages of my life and how that impacted me and others.

As I've said before, I'm a Type A personality. When it comes to my professional work and work ethic, I can get extremely intense and hyper-focused because I always want to do my very best and produce the highest quality results possible. While this can be a positive attribute in many situations, it can also be a negative one. I've most definitely had periods of time in my life when I was drowning in work and not making enough time for my family, friends, and fun. Can you relate? If so, read on!

When I was in college, I could often be found in the library studying for hours and hours on end without taking any real breaks outside of going to the bathroom and grabbing food to eat while I worked. I remember one time when I stayed at the library and studied on a Saturday for seventeen hours straight to prepare for a business law exam! My friends tried to convince me to get a change of scenery and go to lunch or out with them that night, but I was in the zone and couldn't let myself break away.

While I worked full time in corporate marketing at Reebok and simultaneously attended graduate school part time at Boston University, I basically worked all day, went to classes and did homework in the evenings, studied for exams, and worked on group projects during the weekends. Although my husband was in graduate school full time at MIT and worked hard, he often had more free time than I did since I was going to school and working. We were newlyweds at the time, so on many occasions, he had to work hard to convince me to break away from work and school so we could spend quality time together.

When I worked in the digital media industry in Silicon Valley, I often worked over sixty hours each week to keep up with demanding tech clients and internal deadlines. I even kept a crazy work schedule at Google when I was eight months pregnant with my younger son, and my older son was a toddler. I did end up with a promotion right before I left for maternity leave, which was a wonderful reward and seemed to be a strong signal that they wanted me to come back to work after maternity leave. However, it also would have been nice to spend more quality one-on-one time with my toddler before the baby arrived and to have had more downtime with my husband before life got even crazier after we became a family of four.

Looking back, I thought if I worked really hard at that time, I would be able to enjoy my life later. But the harder and harder I worked, the enjoyment that was supposed to happen later just kept getting pushed out further and further. I also thought that achieving success through awards, good grades, and promotions would make me happy and fulfilled, but when I received those things, I often felt empty inside and had a deep longing for my family, friends, and more fun in my life.

Now, don't get me wrong, I certainly had fun with my friends in college, graduate school, throughout my career, and with my family during those years. However, I also experienced periods in my life when I basically had tunnel vision related to work and school, and it took my husband, close friends, or extended family to make me aware of what I was doing and remind me to take breaks, spend more time with them, and get more balance in my life.

Losing all four of my grandparents, a few friends, and other relatives over the years, and living through a global pandemic, has made me even more aware of how short and precious life truly is. We can't always predict what will happen in the future. The greatest gifts we have are the present moments of today, the memories of yesterday, and the hope for what tomorrow may bring. If we're not truly making time to enjoy these treasured moments with those we love, we'll live to regret that later. And no one wants to live, or die, with regrets. Here are four ways to prioritize "The 3 Fs" and ensure that you don't lose sight of what matters most in life.

1. Build time for fun into your daily, weekly, and monthly schedule.

No matter who you are or what you do for a living, honestly, if you don't build time for fun in your life, it may never happen. I strongly encourage you to put fun activities into your daily, weekly, and monthly calendar. I do this myself and encourage my clients to do the same. Whether it's watching your favorite Netflix show, talking to a girlfriend on the phone, going out for a leisurely walk with your significant other, going to the farmers market, ordering takeout, or trying a new restaurant in town, schedule it in. The more fun you're having, the more you'll realize how happy it makes you, and the more you'll prioritize it regularly!

2. Do check-ins with your loved ones on a regular basis.

When we get caught up in the daily grind of life—cooking, cleaning, grocery shopping, working, paying bills, and other responsibilities—we often can lose sight of our feelings and those of our loved ones, because we're just floating from one task to the next. Try to find regular times to do check-ins with your loved ones. You could do it during breakfast, lunch, dinner, before bedtime, or at another time that works for you and your loved ones.

Ensure there aren't any distractions, like the TV and notifications on your phone or other screens, when checking in. You'll also want to make eye contact and give your loved ones your undivided attention, whether you're checking in virtually or in person. Ask them not only how their day is going but also what they're excited about, what might be bothering them, or any other emotions they may be feeling. Share what's happening in all of these areas on your end too.

These check-ins don't have to be extremely long. Spending as little as fifteen minutes at a time could do the trick. Everyone in your immediate and/or extended family will then feel cared for, appreciated, and valued. You may even be able to help them problem-solve or brainstorm an idea, and vice versa.

3. Plan weekend activities, vacations, and short getaways with family and friends.

While some of us are planners and others are not, the more we can spend time on a regular basis thinking about and planning weekend activities, vacations, and other short getaways, the more we'll be reminded of all there is to see, do, and experience in life. Whether you want to do a hike in Yosemite, take a boat ride in Italy, or catch a Broadway show in New York, you gain perspective, something to look forward to, and the ability to see there's more to life than just work, work, and more work. You may already be doing this, and if you are, kudos to you. Keep it up! However, if you're not, or you know someone else who's not, start focusing on it for yourself and others. You may not be able to make every activity or trip happen, but even just going through the motions of thinking about and planning for the future will serve a positive purpose in keeping "The 3 Fs" in the forefront of your mind.

4. Write down your priorities for each season of your life and look at them often.

Whether you're in school, working, and/or raising a family, different seasons in your life call for different priorities. If you can write down and align your goals, choices, and activities with your priorities and core values, you're more likely to make time for "The 3 Fs" and feel fulfilled. For example, if making pancakes for breakfast with your kids is a special bonding activity to do on Saturday mornings in order to align with your values of spending time with your family, be sure to write that down and make the time to do it each week. If doing yoga with your significant other after work a few evenings a week is a way for both of you to manage your stress and spend time together, then write that down and sign up for an ongoing class.

Remember to review these priorities regularly so you can make any necessary changes to them as your life and the lives of your loved ones continue to evolve and change. This review will keep you adapting and responding to what you and others in your life truly need. Remember, "The 3 Fs" are what make life rich and meaningful. Work hard in your career, but continue to push yourself to make time for what truly matters so you can live your most fulfilled life ever!

QUESTIONS

1. What do you like to do for fun, and how can you incorporate fun activities more often into your life?

2. Who matters most to you in your life?

3. How can you spend more time with your family and friends who matter most?

4. What are some dream vacations you want to take, and how can you plan for them in the future?

5. What weekend trips or short getaways might be easy to plan in the coming months?

CHAPTER 11

PURSUE YOUR PASSIONS AND LIVE WITH PURPOSE

WHEN YOU WERE A KID, teenager, and young adult, what subjects and activities were you most passionate about? What got you excited and made you tick? Was it music? Animals? Travel? Fashion? Art? Science? Math? Technology? History? Creative writing? Dance? Sports? Certain charitable causes? As we progress through our lives and careers, and as many of us get married and have children, we get so busy that we often lose sight of these things. We deem them as passions from our youth that no longer have a place in our serious, adult lives.

However, in many cases, these were the very elements of our lives that were authentic to each of us, gave us energy, hope, and purpose, and filled our souls and lit a fire in our bellies! Isn't that what life's all about? Then why should we give up these passions just because we have other priorities and responsibilities? I truly believe our passions can coexist with our jobs, families, and other commitments. We just have to get creative about how best to blend or integrate them. Keeping these passions alive can allow us to live with purpose, play to our strengths, and bring out the best in ourselves and those around us.

According to research studies mentioned in a *Harvard Business Review* article entitled "The Unexpected Benefits of Pursuing a Passion Outside of Work," by Jon M. Jachimowicz, Joyce He, and Julián Arango, pursuing your passions at work can increase your engagement, satisfaction, and performance on the job. However, it can also be extremely beneficial to pursue your passions outside of work. Some of the many benefits include an increase in energy levels and creativity and a decrease in stress and anxiety. These improvements can, in turn, benefit you in your work.

In addition to focusing on your passions, having purpose within your pursuits can further increase the benefits and meaning in your life and the lives of others. So how do you get started? Well, for some people, knowing what to pursue is obvious because it's deeply embedded in them in terms of their natural interests, what they care about, what they talk about regularly, and how they spend their free time. However, for others, it's not so simple. They may be so busy with work and/or their families, that they've buried their passions and sense of purpose because they simply don't have the time. I've had clients on both ends of this spectrum and everything in between. I usually recommend starting with an assessment. Take the time to dig deep and think about the following:

- If you could choose to spend your day doing anything you'd like, what would you do?
- Are there barriers in your life that prevent you from spending your time this way? If so, is this a short-term or long-term challenge, and is there a way to remove this obstacle?
- Are there charitable causes you feel strongly about based on your own life experiences or those you care about?
- What activities make you feel confident and competent?
- What skills do you enjoy and come naturally to you?
- Are you interested in group or solo activities?
- How could you use your passion, talent, or skill to make a positive impact on others?
- Would this pursuit give you purpose and something to look forward to each day?
- Could this pursuit allow you to leave a legacy and create something that will be remembered by others in the future?

As you can see, the types of questions to ask yourself range from lighthearted to deep. They give you the opportunity to think on all levels to truly understand what you're passionate about and to identify what will allow you to live with purpose and make the deepest impact in your life and in the lives of others. Additionally, consider if you want to integrate your passions into your career or pursue them outside of it. There are pros and cons of each path, which are listed below.

Pros of integrating your passions into your work:
- You'll be extremely engaged.
- You'll have a strong purpose.
- You'll enjoy your work and have more freedom in your lifestyle.
- Your work will be aligned with your interests and values.
- You'll be able to play to your strengths and be more confident in your work.

Cons of integrating your passions into your work:
- Your passions may not result in a lucrative or profitable business.
- You may not enjoy your passions as much if they're connected with your work.
- Your passions and interests may change over time, and you may no longer want them to make up your work and career.
- You may not have a clear boundary between your personal and professional life.
- You may experience burnout.

Pros of pursuing your passions outside of work:

- You'll have a nice outlet from work.
- You'll be able to relieve stress through your passions.
- You may be in a different headspace when your passions are for fun versus for work.
- You can enjoy your passions with friends and family.
- Your passions may give you space from work so you can later reengage in your work in a more refreshed and creative way.

Cons of pursuing your passions outside of work:

- You may be too busy and not make the time for your passions when they're outside of work.
- You may miss out on opportunities if your passions could result in a great business idea that could have been especially positive for your career.
- You may feel like something is missing in your professional life if your passions aren't incorporated into your work and are only done outside of it.
- Spending too much time on your passions could result in neglecting your work or other responsibilities in your life.
- You may not be able to bring your strengths into your work if they're only being used through your passions outside of work.

There's obviously a lot to consider here, but the best recommendation I can offer is to simply start. Engage in the passions, interests, and activities that bring you joy and happiness. And if they evolve and change over time, that's okay. You'll be continuously evolving and growing as a person, so your passions could change as your life circumstances change. Conversely, they could end up staying the same if they're deeply embedded passions that have truly shaped you and your life.

A strong example of someone who has consistently followed her passions throughout her life, and has become wildly successful in doing so, is Jennifer Lopez, a first-generation-born Puerto Rican-American singer, dancer, actress, and businesswoman. She is, hands-down, one of my favorite public figures, and she's a truly inspirational boss lady! She has been unapologetically pursuing her passions since the 1990s, and now, in 2021, as a mother, significant other, and professional over fifty years old, she's every bit as strong, vibrant, and relevant as she was back then. She has become one of the most successful women in the entertainment industry today.

She first entered the scene as a "Fly Girl" dancer on the hit show *In Living Color* in 1990 and went on to pursue several movie roles in the 1990s, 2000s, and 2010s, such as *Selena, The Wedding Planner, Maid in Manhattan, Monster-In-Law, The Back-up Plan, What to Expect When You're Expecting,* and *Second Act,* and has become a movie producer. She also has been a successful singer and recording artist with top-performing albums, such as, *On the 6, J.Lo, Rebirth, Love?* and *A.K.A.,* and continues to pursue her love of dance during her concerts and in her music videos. In addition, Jennifer Lopez has been a judge on *American Idol* and *World of Dance*, has her own fashion and skincare lines, gives to many charities she's passionate about, and the list goes on and on.

In a 2018 interview with media company *We Are Mitu,* and according to writer Alyssa Morin, Jennifer Lopez had this to say about pursuing one's passions: "It's about trying different things. It's about finding your passions. It's about not having one passion. Who says you have to have one passion? You can have twenty over a course of a lifetime." As you can see, she's clearly an amazing person and has wonderful insights about finding, pursuing, and leveraging your passions in order to be happy, fulfilled, and successful. I, personally, have always admired her ability to build a career rooted in her passions, since essentially that's what I've been doing with Passion Fit, as it brings me so much happiness and fulfillment.

I encourage you to do the same and discover your inner J.Lo.! In addition to answering the earlier questions about discovering or rediscovering your passions, I invite you to answer the questions below. Having answers to these questions will help you develop a game plan so you can start pursuing your passions today!

QUESTIONS

1. What are your top three to five passions you've had in your life?

2. How can you start incorporating them, or continue to incorporate them, into your life?

3. Would you want them to be a part of your work and career, or would you prefer they stay separate?

4. What benefits will you experience by inviting these passions into your personal and/or professional life?

5. How can you start pursuing your passions today?

CHAPTER 12

THERE'S ONLY ONE YOU IN THIS WORLD!

IN THIS WORLD OF SOCIAL MEDIA, where comparisons, perfectionism, and an obsession with staying youthful seem to be promoted, it's easy to feel less than or not enough. But I want to tell you there's only one YOU in this entire world, and you're beautiful, bold, and brilliant, just the way you are!

If you can tap into and celebrate your own individuality and authenticity and continue to prioritize your physical, mental, emotional, and spiritual well-being, success will be yours in many forms. You'll be able to flourish and be your best self, both personally and professionally. This is what the heart of this book has been all about, and it is what I wish, from the bottom of my heart, for you. So let's dive into this chapter and look at how you can step into your power and fully embrace yourself.

The first step is learning to acknowledge that you're worthy of self-love, which is a topic I feel strongly about. I've experienced firsthand, and have seen for others, what a difference it can make in your life when you put in the work to acknowledge you deserve it and then attain it, versus not believing you're worthy and not having it. According to *Medical News Today*, self-love is a key form of mental health and well-being. By having a deep sense of unconditional self-love, we can have true joy, happiness, and peace in our lives. We also won't have to feel the pressure to be someone we're not and can truly appreciate and enjoy who we are and who we were always meant to be.

However, self-love can be extremely difficult to attain and can often be dependent on or influenced by life circumstances, past events, personality traits, family dynamics, and other natural tendencies. It may take years to truly feel a sense of love for ourselves, but the more we can acknowledge it, prioritize it, and practice it, the better. This could come through regular self-reflection, journaling, taking a break from social media, practicing mindfulness and yoga, and talking to family, close friends, and possibly even a professional. It can also come from reminding ourselves every day of our attributes and being empathetic toward ourselves for our perceived shortcomings.

Different life situations can also test our self-love, such as starting or ending relationships, life transitions, career challenges, failures, family issues, and other personal challenges. We've all been there at one point or another, and these types of situations can be difficult to go through. However, staying authentically true to who we are, loving and believing in ourselves, having confidence in our abilities, having self-respect, and not allowing self-doubt to take over are all ways to allow our self-love to shine through, even in the toughest of times. And while taking these types of actions can be easier said than done, remember to apply them as often as possible because they will truly allow you to pass through various life situations in a much healthier way.

Also, remember we're all human, and we can often be our biggest critics. So, it's imperative that we learn how to consistently silence those critical voices with positive self-talk and self-compassion. The more those voices are nipped in the bud, the less frequently they'll show up. In addition, coupling self-love with ongoing self-care each day can help us create a sense of fulfillment, empowerment, and strength to take on whatever life may bring.

While I feel fortunate to come from an extremely loving and supportive family and have always felt that love and support throughout my life from my parents, grandparents, brothers, sister, husband, kids, in-laws, and extended family, I've still had my struggles at times with self-love and being able to accept my authentic self. Since I'm the youngest in my family, I was compared with my older siblings all the time, whether consciously or unconsciously. These comparisons came from my parents, teachers, sports coaches, family friends, relatives, or others in our community, and people sometimes even had preconceived notions about me upon or before meeting me. And while I didn't mind being compared to my siblings because I'm close to all of them and truly love them with all my heart, as I was growing up, it did make me struggle at times to figure out who I truly was, what I stood for, and what I wanted in life.

It took many years of self-reflection and life experiences to understand my own personality traits, strengths, weaknesses, likes, dislikes, ways of showing up in the world, and approaches to different life situations. It was a complex but necessary journey that continued through my teenage and adult years, during high school, college, within my first several years after college while I worked and attended graduate school, and even when I became a new mom. I finally was able to accept and embrace my true self, rather than question, as I once did, whether I was smart enough, pretty enough, talented enough, or had accomplished enough. I finally realized and have continued to remind myself that I was and still am enough. Period.

Another aspect of stepping into your power and fully embracing yourself is being able to overcome your fears, step out of your comfort zone, and gain confidence, which can also lead to self-love. Being the youngest made these steps difficult for me at times since everyone in my family was extremely protective of me while I was growing up. And because they were all older, they had the wisdom, knowledge, and insights to steer me in the right direction and help me make decisions. While I was grateful for their help, good intentions, and experience, I knew that guidance sometimes made me fearful and hesitant to make my own decisions or try new things because I feared making mistakes or letting people down. As a result, I knew deep down that I needed some independence if I wanted to develop and confidently grow into my own person.

When I considered which job I wanted to pursue after graduating college, I picked a leadership development rotational program with GE, where you move every six months for two years and rotate through different offices, cities, and cross-functional roles, all while taking a curriculum of business courses. It was kind of post-BBA/pre-MBA training. This job took me all over the country, to the Los Angeles, Denver, New York, and San Francisco areas. At first, I was terrified of accepting this job offer because I was born and raised in the Midwest and hadn't yet moved or traveled to many different cities on my own. However, this was the very opportunity I needed to overcome my fears, step out of my comfort zone, and gain some independence from my family. So I accepted the offer and wholeheartedly went into the new job and new life situation with positive intentions, hope, and gratitude.

Looking back at that time, I'll never forget the moment when I was sitting on the floor in my first apartment in the LA area, without any furniture and tons of unopened boxes all around me. I was newly graduated from college and twenty-two years old. I'd just arrived at my apartment from the LAX airport, and I was about to begin living by myself for the very first time. It was my first sense of true independence and liberation, and I remember sitting there in awe, with a huge smile on my face. I knew in that moment that my life as an adult was truly beginning; I could make this experience anything I wanted it to be, and the world was my oyster!

While it was scary, hard, and exhausting at times to experience change so frequently, I'm grateful I did it. I was able to prove to myself and my family that I was capable. I also began to discover my true self through this journey of moving to different cities, living alone in some rotations and with new roommates in others, traveling, working, taking professional courses, and meeting new people. I learned I was strong enough to move to places where I didn't know very many people or anyone at all and still excel at my job, make new friends, and create a happy and productive life for myself. I also became adept at embracing change, which is a hard skill to learn. However, it did get easier with time, practice, and life experience, bringing me one more step closer to developing self-love.

As I discovered, it's important to take on opportunities and challenges, even if you're scared, especially if you know they'll allow you to learn and grow. It won't be easy, but it's worth it in the end and will lead you on an invaluable path of self-discovery.

When I work with my clients, I make it a point to ask lots of questions; understand their challenges, goals, and objectives; and then create customized programs and solutions for them because each client is unique. I try to remind them that there is only one of them in the world, and they need to listen to their own individual needs and wants in order to make positive changes and succeed. I also remind them to love themselves, avoid comparisons with others, overcome their fears, and step out of their comfort zones. These are all areas that take time and effort to work through, since most people struggle in these areas at one point in their life or another.

However, when it all comes together, it's extremely rewarding to see their confidence build, especially when they start to see results and begin to love and believe in themselves and their own transformations more fully. It's one of the many reasons I love the rewarding work I do, and it makes me want to help more and more women achieve these same types of outcomes.

The best way to achieve these types of outcomes is to practice and use helpful tools to begin to truly honor and celebrate yourself. Below are examples of how you can do this for yourself.

1. Tools for self-love:
- **Self-reflection:** Take the time to reflect on your strengths, weaknesses, likes, preferences, and approaches to truly understand what makes you unique.
- **Journal:** Write about your attributes, both to pump you up when you need it and to share empathetic messages with yourself about your perceived short-comings, so you can refer to them when you're not feeling your best and need a pick-me-up.
- **Mindfulness:** Take breaks from social media and take quiet time to yourself to get centered, breathe, and drown out self-doubt, noise, and comparisons from the outside world so you can connect with your true self.
- **Talk to family, close friends, and possibly even a professional:** Talk to those you trust and who know you best or someone who is trained to help you stay focused on your goals, desires, and dreams and can help you overcome the hurdles to achieving them.

- **Self-care:** Take the time on a regular basis to read, take a bath, get a massage, do yoga, listen to music, or do anything that allows you to care for yourself and helps you fill your own cup.

2. Tools for overcoming fears and stepping out of your comfort zone:

- **Take on new opportunities and challenges:** Allow yourself the opportunity to try new things, even if they scare you, so you can stretch, learn, and grow.
- **Be open-minded:** Don't allow your fears to get the best of you. Understand the underlying reasons for those fears, address them as best you can, and keep an open mind when it comes to taking on new opportunities.
- **Have positive intentions:** Practice positive self-talk, expect positive outcomes, work toward them, and believe in yourself and your abilities.
- **Build confidence:** When you overcome your fears and step out of your comfort zone, you'll naturally build your confidence and self-respect, which will increase with every new opportunity you take on.
- **Discover your true self:** Take the time to put yourself in different situations to see how you act and react so you can discover your most authentic self and your true nature.

No matter what's happening in your life, just remember, there's only one YOU in this world, and you don't need to compare yourself to others or ever feel like you're not enough, because you truly are!

QUESTIONS

1. In what ways are you unique?

2. What opportunities scare you?

3. Of those opportunities, which ones are you willing to take on to allow you to step out of your comfort zone?

4. Do you practice self-love and self-care, and if not, how can you start?

5. How can you get more focused on yourself so you don't get caught up in comparisons with others?

CHAPTER 13

"PERFECT" IS A DIRTY WORD

I'LL ADMIT IT, I'm a perfectionist at heart and always have been. While it can allow me to strive for excellence in everything I do to produce the best, high-quality work, it can also be my biggest roadblock to moving forward. And it can make life quite exhausting and challenging at times. I continue to work on letting go of my perfectionism.

If you also deal with perfectionism, I encourage you to consider doing the same because, let's be honest, we're all human, and the concept of perfection isn't realistic or attainable. In my opinion, "perfect" is a dirty word!

Do we want to chase perfection all of our lives, only to be let down time and time again when we fall short of our own unrealistic expectations? Or do we want to try our best in all we do, with a sense of acceptance and peace about things we can't control or that don't go the way we envisioned? The latter will allow us more space to be who we truly are. Then we can go out there and do our thing without worrying so much about having the perfect outcome. We can let the outcome be what it's destined to be. By approaching life in this way, we're all likely to have more fun, enjoyment, learning, growth, and maybe even outcomes beyond our wildest dreams!

Living, working, and raising a family in Silicon Valley, and having worked and studied in other major metropolitan cities across the country, have presented both opportunities and challenges for me. Since I've been surrounded by some of the best and brightest in the world in my professional and academic life, perfectionism has reared its ugly head in many situations—I've felt that pressure over the years. I've experienced times when I felt a sense of defeat, being overwhelmed with my workload while attending graduate school part time and working full time. I've experienced times when I felt imposter syndrome at work in the tech industry, and when I made a mistake, I questioned whether I was good enough at my job. I've experienced times when I questioned my ability to be an entrepreneur, especially when I didn't see growth at the rate I had hoped. And I've experienced times when I felt like a less-than-stellar mom, for instance, when I was too busy to make homemade cookies for a school event and bought them at the grocery store instead. The list goes on and on.

Have you also experienced these types of feelings in different situations in your life? If you have, I understand and empathize with you! However, if you look at some of the examples

I shared, you can see how silly it is to expect perfection in any of these situations. It's normal, natural, and human to feel overwhelmed at times, to make mistakes, to need time for things to grow, and to choose more efficient strategies when life gets busy. I try to remind myself of these truths whenever I feel that sense of perfectionism coming to the forefront of my mind. I invite you to join me and release the chains of perfectionism that often can have such a strong hold on us that we end up getting stuck instead of moving forward.

According to an interview with Alice Boyes, a former clinical psychologist, writer, and author, in the "Women at Work" podcast for the *Harvard Business Review*, professional women are usually more likely than men to suffer from imposter syndrome and anxiety-driven perfectionism, and this is because more men are in leadership roles, and also because women often feel like they have to live up to men's standards and expectations in order to be respected. Also, US society tends to place a high value on perfectionism. These realities create a fear of receiving negative feedback, making mistakes, and letting others down. In addition to the workplace, perfectionism can also come through pressures from the media industry. Whether it's on social media, in movies, on TV, in magazines, or in podcast discussions, there's a lot of focus on women needing to be perfect in their careers, perfect as moms, perfect in how they look, and perfect in being able to "have it all."

In addition to the pressures I've felt in my career and as a mom, I've also felt the pressure to constantly be in shape. Since I'm petite and stand just under five feet tall, throughout my life, I've felt that I have to compensate for my shorter height by having the "perfect" body. While I have a healthy overall approach to exercise and nutrition, because I value my own health and want to ensure I'm walking the talk and being a good role model for my clients, I'll be honest that, at times, I've been hard on myself when it has come to my body image. Thankfully, I'm quite self-aware, so I'm always working on it. I know deep down that being petite isn't cause for shame or something you must compensate for. And luckily, my husband, who's over six feet tall, likes that I'm petite!

While being in shape to be healthy is one thing, being in shape to look good is dangerous because it can result in an unhealthy mindset and unhealthy behavior if we don't deal with it head-on. For that reason, I truly believe in the importance of continuously working on our self-love and self-acceptance, especially as they relate to overcoming perfectionism, and I strive to share that belief with others.

And speaking of others, it's important to my husband and me, especially since we're both recovering perfectionists, to raise our sons to try their best in all they do, but not to be too hard on themselves if they make mistakes. We've already seen them absorb some of our perfectionist tendencies, along with what they pick up from their peers within their schools and sports teams. And while we, of course, want them to have high standards for themselves and strive for excellence in school and sports, it should never be at the expense of their self-esteem, health, and happiness. Ultimately, we want them to enjoy life, work hard, make mistakes, learn from them, and keep growing and going.

One other thought I want to share relates to what happens when perfectionists interact with other perfectionists. I have clients, vendors, and business development partners I work with who are perfectionists too. When perfectionists work with other perfectionists, we see extremely high-quality work, but many, many rounds of revisions and some analysis paralysis. Thankfully, we're all self-aware and know when to pivot or stick with the path we're on and make minor improvements.

If you're looking for ways to overcome your perfectionism, here are four ideas that can help you do just that. These are ones I use myself and work on with my clients:

1. Compete with no one else but yourself.

One of the biggest culprits of perfectionism is competing with others. While the academic, professional, fitness, and sports worlds tend to encourage competition, I believe it's possible to be competitive in a healthy way by simply competing with yourself. When you get too caught up in what others are doing, you may lose confidence and feel desperate to keep up with them.

If you prepare according to a mix of the standards you've been given, along with your own realistic standards, and if you work hard, put your best foot forward, learn, strive for excellence, and have faith, the outcome will be what it's meant to be and will be favorable, no matter what. It's not always about winning, getting a perfect score, or not making a mistake. It's about the learning, growth, and experience along the way and knowing there's enough room in the world for everyone to be successful in their own way.

2. Do your best, but know when good enough is enough.

Perfection is an unachievable goal because, as we know, there's no such thing. Striving for something that doesn't exist can leave you caught in a dangerous circle of defeat, frustration, and disappointment. Believe me, I've been there. And if you've been there, too, you know what an empty feeling it can be when you work hard to achieve something, yet you find yourself wanting more. Nothing is ever good enough in those instances because you keep raising the bar and chasing this elusive goal of perfection.

If you want to be happy, be grateful. Being grateful for your experience, growth, wisdom, and wins, whenever you do achieve them, will allow you to appreciate what you've accomplished and will give you confidence and self-acceptance. And then, perhaps, you won't have to chase perfectionism as much or at all because you'll know that true happiness comes from inside of you and not from your external accomplishments.

3. Complete a project or task now and know you can enhance it later.

If you're a perfectionist, you know how hard it is to finally finish a task, complete a project, or launch a product, because you want to keep making it better and better. However, if it's any consolation, in many cases, you can continue to enhance it even after you complete or launch it. When I worked for Google, one of the core innovation principles we learned, which is publicly known, is the concept of "launch and iterate." Launch a product and keep iterating and making it better and better. It doesn't have to be perfect, and there's so much you can learn from each iteration. This frame of thinking inside Google is one of the many reasons why the company leads in innovation and excellence and is so successful. So the next time you're having a hard time completing a project or task for fear of failure or that it won't turn out perfectly, remember to "launch and iterate"!

4. Give yourself a break sometimes and don't take everything so seriously.

At the end of the day, life isn't perfect, so why on earth do you have to be? Don't let perfectionism take the joy out of your life. Give yourself a break and don't take yourself and everything else so seriously. If you can take a step back and get some perspective on what truly matters, hopefully, you'll realize perfectionism isn't worth sacrificing your happiness. And the imperfections of life can be beautiful in their own right! While everyone has different goals, for most of us, whether we realize it or not, it's not as much about achieving the actual goal as it is about how it makes us feel. And if you sacrifice everything to be perfect and achieve that goal, you may not feel the way you intended—you may even feel empty and depleted inside. So focus on your health, happiness, and well-being, no matter what, and you'll hopefully end up feeling the way you ultimately want to feel, whether or not you achieve the goal. Life is too short to take yourself so seriously, so try your best to take the weight off your shoulders and lighten up! When you realize perfection isn't realistic and robs you of having a healthy and happy life, you'll be able to focus on what matters most: competing with no one but yourself, knowing when enough is enough, completing projects or tasks and enhancing them later, and giving yourself a break and not taking everything so seriously. And if you slip back into your perfectionist ways, just remember: "perfect" is a dirty word!

QUESTIONS

1. Are you a perfectionist or do you have perfectionist tendencies?

2. If so, what are your biggest fears or reasons for wanting to be perfect?

3. How would you feel if you could release the need to be perfect?

4. What can you do to start letting go of perfectionism?

5. If you ever revert to your perfectionist ways, what phrase do you want to keep in mind?

CHAPTER 14

FAIL, FLOURISH, AND FLY!

WHILE FAILURE IS DEFINED in the dictionary as a lack of success, I've learned over time that it's not a lack of success but rather one more step toward success. The more comfortable we can be with failure, the freer we can be to take risks and try new things. When we try new things, we open up our capacity for growth, and that's how we flourish as individuals—and that's when we can truly fly!

I want to challenge you to look at failure in a completely different way than you may have in the past. Redefine it and let it empower you rather than hinder you. This chapter is intended to inspire you and show you how!

According to a January 21, 2016, article in *Entrepreneur* by author Travis Bradberry, entitled "8 Ways Intelligent People

Use Failure to Their Advantage," research studies have shown that the best way to find success in the face of failure is to focus on the desired results, rather than trying not to fail. If we're constantly focused on our fear of failing, we almost fear it into existence. We get anxious, we lose confidence, and we're not able to perform at our best. However, if we're laser-focused with our eyes on the ideal outcomes we want, we'll keep trying different strategies and paths to get to those outcomes or the ones we're destined to achieve. And when we're especially hungry for success, we'll keep working to make it happen and use the failures along the way to our advantage, rather than allow them to cause us to give up.

While Vera Wang, a first-generation-born Chinese-American and a well-respected and world-class bridal gown designer, is a household name today, she experienced her fair share of failures over the years on her way to success. Many people may not know that her original dream was to be an Olympic figure skater, as she started training in figure skating at the age of eight. According to a November 3, 2020, article by ZK Goh in the *Olympic Channel*, Vera Wang competed in the US Figure Skating Championships, but when she tried out for the US Olympics team in 1968, she, unfortunately, wasn't selected. She took that failure and decided to pivot professionally and focus on the fashion industry in the 1970s and 1980s. She held successful roles as the youngest-ever fashion editor at *Vogue* and design director at Ralph Lauren.

When she turned forty years old and was planning her wedding to Arthur Becker, she found a lack of bridal gown options for more mature brides, so she decided to pivot once again in her career and became a bridal gown designer herself. She has now become one of the premier designers in the world, runs a business worth over $1 billion, and has designed wedding gowns for public figures such as Alicia Keys, Victoria Beckham, and Sarah Michelle Gellar. She has also come full circle and designed figure skating costumes for Olympic figure skaters such as Michelle Kwan, Nancy Kerrigan, and others. Talk about taking your failures, pivoting to new career paths, fulfilling needs in the market, and turning them into successes!

Sometimes opportunities can come when you least expect them, and if you put your fear of failure aside, you just never know what might happen and how it might impact you for the rest of your life. This happened to me. It was the spring of 2003, and my husband and I were engaged, working on final plans for our wedding, and getting ready to move across the country from San Francisco to Boston. My husband had been accepted into MIT for his MBA and MS in Engineering, which was the main reason for our cross-country move after our wedding. I was also planning to apply to graduate schools in Boston once we got there and had an offer to transfer from the San Francisco office of my current company, CNET, to their Cambridge office. However, I knew Reebok was headquartered in the Boston area, and I had always thought it would be so amazing to work there if I ever lived in that area. Given my background in fitness and dance, I was a longtime fan of the Reebok brand and products. So, this was my big chance!

Unfortunately, I didn't know a single person who worked at Reebok at that time and didn't know anyone in my professional or personal network who had any ties to the company either. My choices were to apply through their website and have my resume buried under thousands of other resumes or get creative and find another way to apply. So I started doing some research and spent a lot of time looking through their website and reading press releases and industry articles to see if I could find a contact person. In one of the articles, I came across the name of the Chief Marketing Officer (CMO) and also saw his corporate email address at the bottom of the article.

I took my chances and sent him an email explaining that I was a huge fan of Reebok, I had both a fitness and marketing background, I was moving to the Boston area that summer, and I was planning to be in town in a few weeks with my fiancé on an apartment-hunting trip. I asked if I could meet with him for an informational discussion about the company and future opportunities while I was in town. I had no idea if he would ever write back, since this was the CMO of Reebok, for crying out loud! But I gave it a try by sending the email, along with my resume. What did I have to lose? The worst thing that could happen was that he'd never write back, but at least I'd know I tried. And I could always try another strategy or accept the wonderful CNET job offer I already had.

Well, guess what happened next? He emailed me back within one hour and told me he appreciated my strong interest in the company, he liked my background in fitness and market-ing, and he'd be happy to meet with me when I came into town in a few weeks. Wait ... what?! Was this really happening? It was, and I had to pinch myself because I couldn't believe it. I immediately wrote back to him and suggested some dates and times for the informational session.

This time, however, he didn't write back within an hour, a day, or even a week. At that point, I started to get nervous. I knew he was probably a very busy person, but if he said he was able to meet with me, why wouldn't he respond? So once again, I took a chance. After a week, I called the number that was in the auto signature in his email. Unfortunately, he didn't answer, but thankfully, his administrative assistant did. I asked if I could speak to him about an upcoming meeting I was trying to schedule, but she said he was out of the country traveling on business and wouldn't be back for a few weeks.

Given I was heading to Boston in a few weeks for the apartment-hunting trip and needed to get back to my company, CNET, to let them know if I wanted to take their transfer offer or not, I didn't have much time to wait for him to get back from his trip, respond to me, and then figure out a time to meet. So I honestly told her my situation and how much I was hoping to schedule our meeting as soon as possible. She said, "Sure, honey, how does 9:30 a.m. on the tenth sound?" I, of course, said, "Yes, that works!" I locked in that meeting as fast as I could and thanked her for helping me schedule it. A little side note and lesson learned here: always be nice to administrative assistants because they can be of more help than you know.

Finally, it was time for my husband and me to head to Boston for our apartment-hunting trip and my meeting. I had prepared for weeks for this meeting and was ready—extremely nervous, but ready nonetheless! When I first walked into his office and introduced myself, he looked a little confused and said, "I remember your email, but I don't remember scheduling this meeting with you." My stomach dropped, but I quickly told him I had called to schedule the meeting, and since he was traveling out of the country, his administrative assistant scheduled it for me. He said, "Oh, right ... okay ... great." *Whew!*

He ended up doing a formal interview with me that day and asked me some pretty tough questions. Thankfully, I had spent a lot of time preparing, and the interview went well enough that he wanted to schedule additional interviews for me with some VPs and directors in HR, interactive marketing, and women's marketing. I ended up interviewing with six different people over the next few days, then had to wait a few more weeks, and then ... I received an offer for a global interactive marketing manager position about a week before my wedding! I was on top of the world, as I was getting married to the love of my life, embarking on an exciting move to an amazing city, and starting my dream job with a company I had always wanted to work for.

What I loved most about working for Reebok was that it allowed me to combine my professional background in marketing with my personal passions of health, wellness, and fitness. It was the perfect fit for me, and I went on to work at Reebok for two years. I had such an incredible experience working with talented people, and learning, contributing, and growing as a marketing professional. The only reason I ended up leaving the company after two years was because my husband and I knew we wanted to move back to California after graduate school to settle down and start a family. There were also more long-term job opportunities in California for both of us, and Reebok didn't have any full-time positions on the West Coast at that time. However, it was a professional experience I'll never forget, and to this day, I'm so incredibly grateful for the opportunities it afforded me.

I share this story to illustrate the fact that we all have it deep within us to take nothing and turn it into something—if we work hard, believe in ourselves, take a chance, overcome fears of failure, and try. It takes guts and tenacity, but if you want something badly enough, you can strive for it without worrying about the outcome, and if it's meant to be, it will happen. So the next time you want to sign up for a marathon or triathlon, apply for a new job, start your own business, publish a book, take a new class, go back to school, travel around the world, go rock climbing, or whatever it may be, don't be afraid to fail. Take a chance and try because you never know what might happen, and you may just flourish and fly!

QUESTIONS

1. Are you afraid of failure in any aspect of your life?

2. If so, why and what's the worst thing that can happen if you fail?

3. What positive outcomes could you experience if you let go of your fear of failure in this area?

4. Do you have an example in your life when you failed, and if so, how were you able to recover and learn from it and then later succeed?

5. What's one action you can take today toward achieving a goal without worrying about failure?

CHAPTER 15

SISTERHOOD AND COMMUNITY ... YOUR SAVING GRACE

IN LAUNCHING MY COMPANY, Passion Fit, my mission since day one has been to empower women to flourish both personally and professionally through wellness, and my vision has been to create and continue to build both a local and global online wellness community where women can have fun, make friends, feel supported, and be encouraged to achieve their dreams and goals. In the last several years of making my mission and vision a reality, I've seen how powerful our sisterhood and community really are. The women in the Passion Fit community, who take the fitness and dance classes, shop for the activewear, consume the online content, attend the retreats and events, follow on social media, read the blog and newsletters, use the YouTube channel, and become personal and professional development coaching clients, are some of my dearest friends. And in reading this book, you're becoming a wellness-empowered woman who is also part of our Passion Fit community!

I find when you put the time and energy into connecting with others through a community, you feel fulfilled. And what a great feeling it is to form a bond with others through listening, talking, and helping, while allowing them to listen, talk, and help you. I also find relating to and being there for others, in good times and challenging times, allows you to feel mutually understood and not alone.

In many instances, someone has been where you are and can share their reactions, thoughts, suggestions, and advice based on their own experiences. Oftentimes, you can do the same for them. Everyone goes through tough times at one point or another when it comes to raising children, navigating careers and the ups and downs within marriages, dealing with health issues, tending to family needs, and managing finances and other challenging and demanding life circumstances. Having the ability to rely on your community can help get you through those tough times with love and support. Whether you want to connect with two people or twenty-two, find people you trust and with whom you feel a kinship, and then keep building from there.

When it comes to health and wellness, communities can be especially powerful. According to a June 22, 2015, *U.S. News* article by contributor Gloria Caulfield, a healthy community can enhance how we live, work, and play, and can deliver a quality of life that emphasizes health, well-being, and social-connectedness.

From my experience, here are four ways a wellness community can motivate and inspire us all to be healthy and successful in all aspects of our lives.

Accountability: We can feel a sense of accountability to one another to stay the course and show up for scheduled workouts, eat nutritious foods, manage stress, be productive, and practice an overall healthy lifestyle. When we're part of a group, we're more likely to understand the importance of keeping our promises and not letting others or ourselves down. The collective group can help hold everyone accountable and is often more powerful than if we were to go it alone.

Inspiration: When we see others within a community achieving goals and overcoming challenges, we may feel inspired that the same can happen for us. Seeing others succeed can offer hope for our own future success. Inspiration provides us with an emotional connection to each other as well as to our health, well-being, and life in general. That emotional connection is critical for taking action and staying committed, even when times get tough.

Leadership: Wellness communities often have leaders who are trained to understand what others might need to stay healthy and can offer expert feedback and advice. General and specialized group fitness instructors, trainers, nutrition specialists, mindfulness gurus, wellness and life coaches, and more can play a vital role in leading the community in a positive and effective way. The community can learn from such leaders and one another, which can provide a wonderful opportunity for continuous growth and development when it comes to our health, wellness, and life.

Impact: The goal of many communities is to grow, enabling more people to take part and benefit from them. It could be a great opportunity to give back to the community as a whole by recruiting more members and helping others achieve their wellness goals. As the community grows, so does the strength of the collective group, including the knowledge, wisdom, encouragement, learning, and overall opportunity to achieve something bigger than ourselves.

In addition, there's such power in women supporting women and coming together in the spirit of wellness, community, and personal and professional growth and development to connect, learn, share, teach, empathize, show kindness, empower, and become stronger together in all aspects of life. No matter what life may bring, having a community of girlfriends to belong to can truly be your saving grace.

I feel incredibly lucky to have an amazing tribe of women from all the different chapters in my life; they truly motivate and inspire me every day. My tribe consists of my mom, sister, mother-in-law, sisters-in-law, cousins, aunts, nieces, girlfriends from school, neighbors, fellow moms in our local school community, and professional contacts. Many of these women are part of the Passion Fit community, which is really special.

These women have been with me during all the big and small milestones throughout my life. They were my study buddies in school. They were part of my cheerleading and dance team squads. They were and still are my sorority sisters. They were my roommates in and after college. They were with me during the nights out when I met and later started dating my husband. They were there to celebrate my engagement. They were shoulders to cry on when my grandparents passed away. They were bridesmaids and readers in my wedding. They were there when I found out I was pregnant with each of my sons. They threw bridal and baby showers for me. They were there when I walked away from my corporate career and launched Passion Fit. They've brought over meals when my husband or I have been sick. They've been there to bring one or both of our boys home from school, soccer, or basketball practice when we had a schedule conflict. They've been there as my confidence-boosters when I've struggled to balance work and motherhood. The list of the ways these women have been there for me is endless. I don't know what I'd do or who I'd be without them. I love them with all my heart, and I'm always there to support each and every one of them throughout their lives!

I now invite you to reflect on the communities and women in your life and answer the following questions. I hope this activity will allow you to realize the impact they've had on you and you've had on them!

QUESTIONS

1. What does community mean to you?

2. What are the most important communities you're a part of in your personal and professional lives?

3. Who are the women who have had the most profound impact on you throughout your life?

4. Do you have a wellness community to keep you motivated in your health and wellness?

5. What can you do to support other women and to continue to stand for gender equality and empowerment, both inside and outside of the workplace?

CONCLUSION

NOW, MORE THAN EVER, women need to be brave, strong, healthy, and empowered. In the last several years, we've experienced the Me Too and Time's Up movements, we continue to fight the gender pay gap and other inequalities in the workplace, and we continue to express the need for more diversity and inclusion. We've also been hit by a global pandemic, which has caused many women to have to step out of the workforce due to conflicts with work and childcare needs.

According to an article by Julia Boorstin in *CNBC*, a "Women in the Workplace" research study was conducted in 2019 by the consulting firm McKinsey and Company and an organization named LeanIn.Org. In this study, 73 percent of women reported experiencing discrimination in the workplace on a daily basis. In addition, only 21 percent of women were in the C-suite, and only one in twenty-five women in the C-suite was a woman of color. Also, according to the *latest*

"Women in the Workplace" research study conducted in 2020 by McKinsey and LeanIn.Org, one in three women considered downshifting their careers or leaving the workforce altogether because of the pandemic.

I wrote *The Wellness-Empowered Woman* throughout 2020 and into 2021. How are these still major issues for women in the workplace twenty years into the 21st century? So much work still needs to be done to create positive change and close these gaps. And guess who needs to be leading the charge for that change to happen? Women, of course! Luckily, we now have our first female Vice President of the United States, and no matter where you may stand politically, Kamala Harris will indeed be a prominent figure in leading this charge for all women.

In order to lead in the most impactful and game-changing way, we have a responsibility to be at our best. And in order to be at our best, we have to be mentally, physically, emotionally, and spiritually healthy. In my mind, wellness is at the center of it all. Women need each other, and we need wellness in order to rise up, not only for ourselves and out of respect for the generations that came before us, but now more than ever, for the generations that will come after us. These girls are or will be our daughters, granddaughters, nieces, and mentees. They're depending on us to be educated, healthy, balanced, mindful, passionate, strong, kind, giving, tenacious, and resilient. If they see us living as wellness-empowered women, they'll have a roadmap to follow when they become women.

We need to set an example for the next generation of boys too. These boys are our sons, grandsons, nephews, and mentees. If we can teach them to be healthy and educated and to treat women with respect, as equal and true partners in life, we'll have done something significant for society and the world. Being a mom of two boys, I feel especially passionate about teaching my boys to treat girls fairly, equally, and respectfully. My husband feels the same way and is a wonderful supporter of women's empowerment and a fantastic role model for our sons.

Positive change starts with each and every one of us in our homes, within our families, in the workplace, and in our communities. For this reason, my focus with each of my clients is on the whole person. It starts with the woman herself, but also includes her significant other, her children and family as a whole, and her personal and professional life. When we can come together as women, we can truly do anything. We're unstoppable, individually and collectively. We're wellness-empowered women!

A SPECIAL MESSAGE TO YOU, THE READER

WELL, WE'VE COVERED A LOT OF GROUND together throughout this book, haven't we?! I'm truly honored and so grateful you found this book and have been introduced to Passion Fit's philosophies on wellness and its deep connection to both personal and professional development and success.

My sincere hope is that *The Wellness-Empowered Woman* has touched your heart and will positively impact your life in some way. While each of us has our own unique wellness journey and life path to follow, I feel we can always find common ground and relate to one another as busy women trying to be our best selves—to make a positive impact on our families, friends, communities, companies, and the world around us.

Thank you for allowing me to be a small part of your journey. I would love for us to stay connected, so please be sure to visit my website at passionfit.com and connect with me and my community on social media. Also, I invite you to send me an email at reena@passionfit.com and schedule a free fifteen-minute introductory call so I can learn more about you and we can determine how Passion Fit might help you reach your goals. I'd love to be a part of what comes next for you!

Whether this is the beginning of your wellness journey or you have been on this journey for a while, you have the ability, with focused intention and commitment, to continue on the path of a wellness-empowered woman. Cheers to you on your journey, along with my most heartfelt wishes for love, joy, peace, happiness, good health, prosperity, and success in your life, always!

With Love,
Reena Vokoun

ABOUT THE AUTHOR

REENA VOKOUN, founder and CEO of Passion Fit, is an author, TEDx speaker, media spokesperson, certified health and wellness expert, personal and professional development coach and consultant, content creator, and marketer.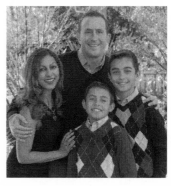

Reena graduated with a BBA in Marketing and Management from the University of Wisconsin-Madison and an MS in Advertising and Communications from Boston University. She spent years in marketing, sales, and business development for Google, Yahoo, Reebok, CNET, GE, and Grokker.

Today, she serves companies, nonprofits, universities, schools, and the media through Passion Fit products, services, and content on fitness, nutrition, mindfulness, and work-life balance.

Reena is featured as a TV health contributor on Fox KTVU news and NBC California Live, speaks to companies such as Microsoft, Google, and Amazon, is a newspaper health columnist, and writes for *Thrive Global, Shape, Working Mother,* and her own blog. She's on the Entrepreneurship Advisory Board for the University of Wisconsin-Madison and is a Women in Management Facilitator for Stanford University.

Reena is a wife, mom, and first-generation-born Indian-American who lives in California. Visit passionfit.com to learn more about how you can connect with Reena and her amazing Passion Fit community.

ACKNOWLEDGMENTS

WRITING THIS BOOK has been both an enormous and rewarding undertaking, and I couldn't have done it without the support of the following incredible people.

Book Team:

Thank you to my amazingly talented publishing consultant, Kirsten Jensen; editor, Donna Mazzitelli; proofreader, Jennifer Jas; book designer, Victoria Wolf; and publishing advisor, Polly Letofsky, for their endless support in helping me bring my book to life. They've made this process fun and engaging, and I've loved every minute of working with them. Also, thank you to my fellow author and wellness professional, Cheryl Ilov, for her belief in me as a writer and for introducing me to this team. I sincerely appreciate it.

Thank you to my wonderful PR and book marketing experts, including Kristi Dosh, Vicky Lynch, and the rest of their amazing team. I sincerely appreciate their incredible industry knowledge and efforts to help me get the word out about the book. I'm so lucky to have them in my entrepreneurial tribe, and I truly love working with them.

Thank you to my web experts, Deb Wise and Vanja Drobina, for their excellent web development and design work for the book. Their technical support was incredibly helpful, and I'm so thankful for them.

Thank you to my photographer, Alex Johnson, for his artistry in bringing my vision of the book cover to life. His talent and creativity are exceptional, and he's always a pleasure to work with.

Thank you to my lawyer, Claire Kalia, for her guidance and support in the trademark and copyright aspects of publishing this book. Her knowledge and work are truly incredible, and she always has thorough answers to all of my legal questions and needs.

Thank you to my original agent, Linda Konner, for her efforts at the start of my writing and publishing journey and her support throughout. I learned so much about the publishing industry through her many years of experience.

Thank you to Jennifer Dulski, Bonita Stewart, Lexi Reese, Meredith Momoda, Mary Oleksy, Meredith Bodgas, and Kristi Dosh for providing advanced reader reviews for the book. They're all talented and inspiring female leaders whom I've worked for or with throughout my career, and I'll be forever grateful for their positive influence on me.

The journey to bring *The Wellness-Empowered Woman* into the world has only just begun. I know many other people and teams will help in the days, weeks, months, and years ahead, and I thank you in advance for your support and expertise as we continue to spread the word for this labor of love.

Professional, Academic, and Charitable Networks:

Thank you to all of my brilliant former and current managers, mentors, colleagues, industry peers, cross-functional teams, and business development partners from all the companies where I've worked—Google, Yahoo, Reebok, CNET, GE, and Grokker—and with my own company at Passion Fit. They've helped shape my career, and I wouldn't be where I am today without all of them.

Thank you to all of my teachers, coaches, alumni boards and councils, alumni relations teams, professors, and career development counselors at Kettle Moraine High School, University of Wisconsin–Madison, and Boston University. They created the foundation for my academic experience, and they've turned me into a lifelong learner.

Thank you to the smart and kind Women in Management facilitators and students at Stanford University for enriching my personal and professional development and experiences. I'm honored to be part of such a special group of female leaders and change-makers.

Thank you to the powerhouse organizer, speaking coach, video production team, event planning team, and fellow speakers at TEDxDelthorneWomen. I'm grateful for our life-changing experience on that TEDx stage together, and I love the personal and professional support we continue to have for one another.

Thank you to the managers and teams at the Leukemia and Lymphoma Society Woman of the Year fundraising campaign. I took on this charitable endeavor while I was simultaneously writing this book. Their support meant so much during that special time.

Friends:

Thank you to all of my sweet and best girlfriends from high school, college, my sorority, graduate school, work, moms and significant others groups, my boys' school and sports groups, neighborhood groups, and the entire Passion Fit community. They all know who they are. I treasure their friendship and sisterhood so much, and I look forward to creating more memories together with them and our families in the future. I love them all, and they'll forever hold a special place in my heart.

Family:

And last but certainly not least, thank you from the bottom of my heart to my amazing husband and precious sons for their constant love, support, and faith in me. They're my rock, my heart and soul, and my whole world. I'm so blessed and grateful for having them in my life, and I love them very much. Thank you also to my incredible parents, late grandparents, brothers, sister, in-laws, nieces, nephews, aunts, uncles, and cousins. They're my foundation, and they've shaped me into the woman I am today. I'm everything I am because of all of them, and I love and cherish them with every ounce of my being.

NOTES

Chapter 2 – What's Your Gut Telling You?

1. Susan Krauss Whitbourne, PhD, "When Should You Trust Your Intuition?" *Psychology Today*, June 9, 2015, https://www.psychologytoday.com/us/blog/fulfillment-any-age/201506/when-should-you-trust-your-intuition.

2. American Psychological Association, "2017 Stress Statistics," *The American Institute on Stress*, https://www.stress.org/daily-life.

3. Kelly Bulkeley, PhD, "Intuition and Dreams: Four Questions to Ask of Each Dream," *Psychology Today,* January 8, 2018, https://www.psychologytoday.com/us/blog/dreaming-in-the-digital-age/201801/intuition-and-dreaming-four-questions-ask-each-dream.

4. Sarah DiGuilio, "Your weird dreams actually make a lot of sense (according to neuroscience and psychology)," interview of Robert Stickgold, PhD, and Associate Professor of Psychiatry at Harvard Medical School's Center for Sleep and Cognition, *NBC News BETTER*, September 27, 2018, https://www.nbcnews.com/better/pop-culture/ your-weird-dreams-actually-make-lot-sense-accord- ing-neuroscience-psychology-ncna913436.

Chapter 3 – Balance, Integration, or Whatever You Want to Call It!

1. Eric Garton, "Employee Burnout Is a Problem with the Company, Not the Person," *Harvard Business Review*, April 6, 2017, https://hbr.org/2017/04/ employee-burnout-is-a-problem-with-the-company- not-the-person.

Chapter 4 – Your Genes Don't Have to Determine Your Jeans

1. Deepak Chopra, MD, and Rudolph E. Tanzi, PhD, *Super Genes* (New York: Harmony Books, 2017).

2. BJ Fogg, PhD, *Tiny Habits: The Small Changes That Change Everything* (Boston: Houghton Mifflin Harcourt, 2019).

Chapter 5 – The Calm Before the Storm?

1. Seth J. Gillihan, PhD, "How Often Do Your Worries Actually Come True?" *Psychology*

Today, July 19, 2019, https://www.psycholo-
gytoday.com/us/blog/think-act-be/201907/
how-often-do-your-worries-actually-come-true.

2. Anxiety and Depression Association of America,
    https://adaa.org/understanding-anxiety/
    facts-Statistics.

3. Harvard Medical School, *Harvard Health
    Publishing,* published April 2009 and updated
    October 13, 2020, https://www.health.harvard.edu/
    mind-and-mood/yoga-for-anxiety-and-depression.

4. National Center for Complementary and Integrative
    Health (NIH), "Meditation: In Depth," https://www.
    nccih.nih.gov/health/meditation-in-depth.

Chapter 6 – No Matter What Else Is Going On, Keep Moving!

1. Harvard School of Public Health, *The Nutrition
    Source,* "Staying Active," https://www.hsph.
    harvard.edu/nutritionsource/staying-active/.

2. American Heart Association, "Why is physical
    activity so important for health and well-being?"
    https://www.heart.org/en/healthy-living/fitness/
    fitness-basics/why-is-physical-activity-so-import-
    ant-for-health-and-wellbeing.

Chapter 7 – Sleep On It ... Tomorrow Will Be a New Day

1. Centers for Disease Control and Prevention, "Sleep and Sleep Disorders: Data and Statistics," https://www.cdc.gov/sleep/data_statistics.html.

2. Joe Leech, MS, medically reviewed by Atli Arnarson, BSc, PhD, "10 Reasons Why Good Sleep Is Important," *healthline,* February 24, 2020, https://www.healthline.com/nutrition/10-reasons-why-good-sleep-is-important.

Chapter 8 – Expect the Unexpected and Get Ready to Fire on All Cylinders!

1. Naz Beheshti, "10 Timely Statistics About the Connection Between Employee Engagement and Wellness," *Forbes*, January 16, 2019, https://www.forbes.com/sites/nazbeheshti/2019/01/16/10-timely-statistics-about-the-connection-between-employee-engagement-and-wellness/?sh=31d94f2222a0.

2. The Energy Project, https://theenergyproject.com/.

Chapter 9 – Hey Honey, What's for Dinner?

1. US Department of Health & Human Services (HHS.gov), President's Council on Sports,Fitness & Nutrition, "Facts and Statistics: Nutrition," https://www.hhs.gov/fitness/resource-center/facts-and-statistics/index.html.

2. Claire Sissons, reviewed by Jillian Kubala, MS, RD, "What is the average percentage of water in the human body?" *Medical News Today,* May 27, 2020, https://www.medicalnewstoday.com/articles/ what-percentage-of-the-human-body-is-water.

Chapter 11 – Pursue Your Passions and Live With Purpose

1. Jon M. Jachimowicz, Joyce He, and Julián Arango, "The Unexpected Benefits of Pursuing a Passion Outside of Work," *Harvard Business Review*, November 19, 2019, https://hbr.org/2019/11/ the-unexpected-benefits-of-pursuing-a-passion-out-side-of-work.

2. Alyssa Morin, "We Sat Down With Jennifer Lopez to Talk About Her Latest Movie 'Second Act' And Why It's Important to Remain Loyal to Your Dreams," December 13, 2018, https://fierce.wearemitu.com/ entertainment/jennifer-lopez-told-us-the-surprising-thing-her-parents-did-to-shape-her-whole-life-and-career/.

Chapter 12 – There's Only One YOU in This World!

1. Ana Sandoiu, fact-checked by Jasmin Collier, "Why self-love is important and how to cultivate it," March 23, 2018, https://www.medicalnewstoday.com/ articles/321309.

Chapter 13 – Perfect Is a Dirty Word

1. Alice Boyes, "Women at Work" podcast, *Harvard Business Review*,https://hbr.org/podcast/2018/10/perfect-is-the-enemy.

Chapter 14 – Fail, Flourish, and Fly!

1. Travis Bradberry, "8 Ways Intelligent People Use Failure to Their Advantage," *Entrepreneur*, January 21, 2016, https://www.forbes.com/sites/travisbradberry/2016/04/12/8-ways-smart-people-use-failure-to-their-advantage/?sh=521feb124489.

2. ZK Goh, "Vera Wang talks about her Olympic ambitions," November 3, 2020, https://www.olympicchannel.com/en/stories/news/detail/vera-wang-talks-about-her-olympics-ambitions/.

Chapter 15 – Sisterhood and Community ...
Your Saving Grace

1. Gloria Caulfield, "Health by Design: the Impact of Community on Wellness," *U.S. News*, June 22, 2015, https://health.usnews.com/health-news/blogs/eat-run/2015/06/22/health-by-design-the-impact-of-community-on-wellness.

Conclusion

1. Julia Boorstin, "One of the biggest reasons women aren't getting ahead at work, according to a new survey," *CNBC*, October 15, 2019, https://www.

cnbc.com/2019/10/15/biggest-reasons-women-ar-ent-getting-ahead-at-work-per-lean-in.html.

2. McKinsey and Company and LeanIn.Org, "Women in the Workplace 2020" research study, https://www.mckinsey.com/featured-insights/diversity-and-inclusion/women-in-the-workplace#.

Made in the USA
Middletown, DE
25 June 2021